"This is a raw, emotionally honest look into teen depression (and by extension, serious depression as a whole). If you want simple answers and certainty, I suggest you look elsewhere, but if you want an unflinchingly honest account of the agony of being a teen without hope, or the difficult (yet rewarding) process of recovery, then know that you've found it!"

JOANNA WESTON, Life Coach

"Suicide Escape captures my torment as a teenager, the joy I've found as an adult and the path between those two worlds in a compelling, thought-provoking drama that is a must read for struggling youth, their families and friends, and anyone battling depression."

KIMMIE FETZER, Certified Nutritionist/Syndicated Radio Host

"Told from the perspectives of a young woman ready to take her life and an old man facing his own mortality, *Suicide Escape* contains easy-to-read, beautiful messages delivered with twists to keep the reader engaged. Having worked on a crisis hotline, the emotions, fears and struggles are spot on."

JENNIFER BRUNDIGE, former Crisis Hotline staff

"As an advocate for teen depression and suicide awareness who has dealt with suicide in my family, *Suicide Escape* brings to life the misunderstood, complex struggle faced by victims of depression. The story, which blurs the line between reality and fiction, also opens minds to the value and purpose of each life."

TANNER SNIDER, Teen Mental Health Awareness Advocate

Suicide
Escape

Mike Bushman

AltFuture Publishing
NAPERVILLE, ILLINOIS

Ordering Information:
Special quantity purchase discounts are available for mental health
agencies, educational institutions, associations and others. For de-
tails, contact:

AltFuture Publishing
932 Commons Road
Naperville, IL 60563

Cover Photograph: ©andreiuc88/Shutterstock
Cover Design: Mike Bushman
Book Layout ©2013 BookDesignTemplates.com

Suicide Escape / Mike Bushman -- 1st ed.
ISBN 978-0-9883369-7-1

Dedicated to Raymond Michael Umbdenstock for displaying humility, humor and hard work, and to Lucille Bushman for demonstrating selflessness, faith and unconditional love, throughout each of their remarkable lives.

Will There
Is There
Can There
Should There
Ever Be

Enough Hope
Dreams
Opportunity
Reason
To Supplant

Such Pain
Anger
Sorrow
Misery
Now Threatening

My Desires
Moments
Aspirations
Successes
And Future

There Should
There Can
There Is
There Will
Ever Be

Foreword

For more than fifteen years I had known Mike from somewhat of a distance to be this intelligent, professional man with kind eyes and engaging presence who loves nature and writing. Only recently, after my own personal struggles, did I come to understand Mike's past experience with suicide and depression. It was surprising—and comforting at the same time—to know that this accomplished and respected man had similar battles with depression and self-worth.

Mike discusses many of his own personal experiences in *Suicide Escape*. As it is for the character Clarissa, sharing one's story is among the hardest, but also most fulfilling methods of dealing with depression, suicidal thoughts or attempts. Equally as important are kindness, availability, human connection and belief that someone cares about you. Throughout the book, you can see Clarissa's positive transformation simply because someone took time to care.

After my first suicide attempt, I thought that I needed some grand life change to kick-start my road to recovery. So I left an eleven-year career and abruptly (practically in the night) left a relationship. A year later, I had my second suicide attempt. This time, still thinking I needed some type of extreme recovery measure, I went to volunteer in Africa. A few months later, I was at the brink of self-destructing—again. It was then when I called a friend and talked about how I felt. I started talking about it to many of my close friends and family for the first time. I shared my story. I asked for help. It was through those moments that I realized I didn't need dramatic action to begin a successful recovery. I needed positive connections. I needed to relish in my morning smile. I needed to stay present and be true to myself. I needed to take one day at a time.

It's interesting how life works. When Mike asked me to write the foreword for *Suicide Escape*, I was, although honored, a little taken aback. I'm not a well-known figure or even a writer for that matter. I began to research how to write a foreword. After a few articles, I came across the line, "If you're writing a foreword, congratulations, it's because you have accomplished something." It's true. I did. Today, two years after my second suicide attempt, I have positive relationships and an amazing partner. I have a strong start to a clearly needed not-for-profit. I want to get up every morning. I always hope to see another day.

Mike's attention and dedication to personal connection and kindness, both in his personal life and in this book, are to be admired. Whether you are struggling personally or know someone who is, you will most certainly connect with a character in *Suicide Escape.*

Carly A. Jacobson
FOUNDER, The C.A.R.L. Project

Clarissa's Note

IT TURNED OUT THAT CLARISSA'S SWEET, fragile soul had been cloaked in a veneer of toughness and independence practically since birth. By the time John Coleman relayed his stories about his daughter, I found little of what he had to say about Clarissa surprising.

A second of inattention left John Coleman chasing down Clarissa after he spotted his then five-year-old new swimmer in mid-jump off a three-meter springboard. The next morning, after an unusually heavy rain, John found Clarissa outside on the driveway picking up worms and gently placing them back where she had decided each must reside.

John said he remembered those particular events because it was the first time he realized that life with Clarissa situated him on a continuous pendulum swing between heartwarming pride and heartbreaking fear.

Clarissa had been daddy's little girl; in many ways the boy the Colemans had hoped to add to their family when they decided to have a third child. When John went to the shooting range, Clarissa was usually his lone company. She was the only one of the girls who enjoyed going to work with John on the many Saturdays he spent trying to optimize his latest waste recycling separation gadget. Clarissa, though, spent most of her time at the lab creating sculptures out of spare parts and garbage strewn around his lab.

John required all three girls to join him for survival training weekends as he increasingly feared for his family's safety, but only Clarissa flourished in the outdoors. As Clarissa careened into her teenage turmoil years, she frequently took off alone on all-day wilderness excursions. Each time, her parents panicked in the hours between when she departed under pretense of going to a friend's house and when she was finally tracked down off trail in the vicinity of Humphreys Peak or another nearby wilderness area.

Only Clarissa's proficiency with a tranquilizer gun—and more recently with an odd-looking rifle John had designed and built—had kept them from always sending the authorities after her when she snuck out and traveled too far to reach quickly. John chased her down many times, tracking Clarissa either with police help through the Lifelink mobile devices common to daily life in 2041 or by using an internet satellite search program at substantial expense. The Colemans never figured out how to punish Clarissa appropriately to keep her from just taking off. When grounded, Clarissa would isolate herself from everyone, disappearing inside the house for long enough that the rest of the family often forgot to check on her. All too often she was long gone by the time they began searching for her. When, instead of grounding, the Colemans took her Lifelink as punishment, Clarissa would sneak out into the woods or nearby canyons or mountains and the Colemans were forced to turn to costly satellite tracking to find her.

In the last few years and particularly in the last few months, John Coleman said he would have given anything to recapture moments of warmth with Clarissa to replace the constant fear barrage that pounded away at his conscience as she isolated herself and became increasingly sullen. Her once-confident disposition had been wilting for years and now seemed completely shredded. Signs of happiness had sunk from occasional to sporadic to nearly nonexistent. John felt helpless to intervene.

Had I really known Clarissa when I first read her suicide note, scrawled out in pencil and shoved inside her clothes in case anyone found her body, I wouldn't have even noticed the destructive impact of autocorrect on her writing skills. Instead, I would have borne some of the soul shattering that John clearly felt in his nearly daily panic.

"ive had enough already. i mean, seriously. people hatin me. callin me stupid, snake hole, skeleton and way way worse. everybody dyin around me. grandpas dead. sarahs dead. nobody knows im alive or even cares. assholes at school are alive and smilin and happy and tellin me im not worth wastin their oxygen. their oxygen. like i dont deserve any. at least theyre honest i guess. my friends abandoned me. great friends huh. thanks for abandoning me girls. you know who i mean. seriously how much am I supposed to just take and take and take and take.

"i just cant do it anymore so i wont. its better this way. its not like anyones gonna care, but in case someone finds my body before its all chewed up and turned into scat, let anyone who asks know that im relieved its over and done with and i dont have to wake up every morning dreading how fucking miserable im gonna be again and whos gonna rip on me in front of everyone, or whos gonna trip me or shove me or grab at me. its weird, but those arent even the worst days. the worst days are when nobody even sees me, even knows im alive or cares. imagine being surrounded by a thousand

people and still being completely utterly alone. aban-
doned. empty. thats my life now. well, it was anyway.

"youre lucky i hate my life more than other people. i
coulda done it too if i really wanted to hurt people, but
then id be an even worse person than the people who
make me sick. i know how to shoot. i coulda gotten a
bunch of people but id still feel terrible. and i dont
want to hurt people because i know what its like to be
hurt all the time. this way, no ones in pain anymore. its
probably the right thing dont you think. i dont wanna
burn in hell and i know id get sent there if I killed
other people. thats where i woulda ended up, always in
the worst place possible. this way, maybe ive gotta shot
of goin if there is a heaven. i mean look at how many
lives i saved gettin rid of mine. thats a lot of people to
save for anyone. and if there isnt a heaven or hell then
im just gone and nothin hurts anymore. anyway tell my
parents and sisters im sorry i got found. id just as soon
they just figured i ran away than have to know im dead
but if you see this it is what it is i guess.

"at least i dont hurt anymore. sorry."

No teenager should have to feel lingering pain that
reaches that depth. For that matter, neither should
anyone else.

2

Meeting Clarissa

I WAS CATCHING MY BREATH on a tree stump just below the Humphreys Peak tree line when I first spotted Clarissa, bent over in a remote spot well off trail and not even looking around to see if anyone could see her.

More than halfway through a long day of hiking, I hunched over on a long-felled tree trunk, catching my breath, rehydrating and chomping a chocolate orange fruit and fiber bar when my eyes were drawn away from the stark, steep white hills that served as monuments to all who ascended as far as I had come that day. While reveling in a view too simple to be art but too dramatic and majestic to be anything else, motion just hundreds of yards away grabbed my attention.

It was awkward, stilted motion, but enough to command my attention. Almost instantly, I felt compelled to find out what or who else would be up here, removed from the hiking trails that most follow faithfully either to avoid getting lost or to avoid trampling on elements of nature that recover slowly, if ever.

It didn't take long to rule out any animals that could pose a physical threat. Few of the most threatening fauna find food at a tree line more than 11,000 feet above sea level. While the form moved gawkily, it still appeared to move with purpose—human purpose my curiosity wouldn't allow me to ignore. A person this far off trail almost certainly would have come here to be alone. I moved closer anyway, finally getting close enough to realize that the form was a woman. I watched intently as she stood up, picked up a long, thick wooden stick, set it back into the ground and bent back over it.

I couldn't tell initially that she was only a teenager, younger than the children of my children. I like to assume I was drawn to Clarissa because the way she was acting just didn't seem right. It's funny how instincts take over our bodies at times, pushing an old man with high blood pressure and countless unwanted aches out of exhaustion into action, even more than halfway through a long hike.

I am by no means fearless. But the idea of death is far past frightening and approaches in an accelerated march in any case. I never guessed that I would have lived to see this year. Perhaps, I thought, my life's challenges had as a purpose preparing for this test of every ounce of my humanity.

I certainly would not have expected to be alive today thinking back to the summer of 1979, when I woke from a drug- and alcohol-induced nap—I'll call it a nap, anyway—along the metal ridge surrounding a water tower a few towns over from my home. I don't remember how I got up there, but my dealer-friend thought it was hysterical to watch the drunk and stoned little freshman climb up the water tower steps to reach the exterior walkway that ran a rim around the bulbous part of the tower.

This friend, who had become my dealer at about the time we discovered and started picking a wild-growth pot field in West Chicago, later told me he boosted me up so I could pull down the ladder to get started. He bolted when it looked like I would fall off during the climb up the metal-ladder steps. The last he saw me was as I tried to push open the metal floor hatch to climb up to the rim. This convenient stand-in for a friend didn't want to be around to take the blame when I fell.

But this temporary friend, who I'll leave unnamed since he may have gone on to respectable life, came back later to see what happened. I don't know if I fell asleep before or after he left, because to this day I don't remember climbing up. But I do remember what it felt like to regain consciousness looking down through the metal grates to ground that seemed a long distance removed, particularly for someone who didn't even enjoy standing high up on a ladder. I had enough of a fear of heights that I felt my stomach convulse, whether out of simple natural reaction or substance-induced nausea wasn't quite clear.

At fourteen back then, I was already at a point where I really didn't care if I lived to see the next day, or hour, or even minute. Every moment of life simply hurt. The pit of my stomach often felt a depth of pain I only later recalled being equal to the agony of watching my father's cancer-riddled body breathe in its last bit of oxygen. I didn't realize how fortunate I had been to reach fourteen with so little experience at dealing with death. With this depression, this shredding pounding a near constant at that age, I didn't often think about whether I wanted to die. Instead, I thought about how to die, when, and whether I could make my body disappear so no one would have to actually know.

It's not that I didn't have a family who loved me. Looking back, I realize I was blessed, particularly considering the crap excuses for families many must endure. I look at kids who survive continuous abuse, neglect and drug-addicted parents—or who live in surroundings containing all the physical threat of a war zone with no commensurate opportunity for glory—and wonder what it was that made me think I had a horrific life destined only for failure. But, over well more than a year, that feeling beat at me to create a relentless barrage of self-loathing, broken by only temporary respites of slightly more tolerable but still intense self-doubt.

The reality is that I didn't want to hurt my family. But I hated myself and couldn't see any chance that life would get better. I just couldn't take how much it hurt to be alive, knowing, or at least thinking, my misery would just compound itself into eternity.

On the first day of freshman football, I measured in at four feet eleven inches. On as full of a stomach as I could muster, I weighed in at a staggering ninety-eight pounds. With physical presence like that, and zero previous football experience, you can imagine I wasn't a star athlete. Even use of the word athlete to describe me was a stretch. Perhaps for giggles but more likely because there just weren't that many boys on the freshman team at Geneva High School in Illinois, the coach would have me practice at offensive tackle some days. I would line up across from the true stud defensive lineman on the team. At double my weight, he would regularly pound me into the turf milliseconds after the snap. Every once in a while, I would succeed in chopping at his knees. On the occasions my chop block worked, he would get back up and then throw me into the turf angry that I cut his legs. "Block like a man, you wuss," he would bark.

After many weeks of this beating, I met the varsity team physician/dealer. He wasn't actually a doctor, trainer or anything close; just a varsity player with spare time to acquire and distribute pain-reduction therapies. By the end of the season, I was inhaling an occasional dose of weed therapy. As bad as I was at football to start the season, I was even worse by the end. I don't blame the coaches in any way for my pot and hash use. I would have found a reason to start regardless. It seemed the cool thing to do and I was eager to erase one of few sources of developmental delay I thought I controlled compared to some of my Catholic elementary school classmates.

By the time the next summer came around, after my freshman year, I had been getting high for a stretch already, though I was doing most of my smoking in the back alley behind a restaurant where I bussed tables or stopped off somewhere on the way home from work. I'd started wearing cowboy boots under wide-flare jeans to school, providing a convenient place inside each boot to store some of my stash for far less common midday use. I slowed down on the weed a bit during tennis season that freshman year. Having recently crossed the five-foot threshold, I played doubles on the sophomore tennis team with a sophomore partner who would turn to me at crucial points in almost every match and spout his words of motivational wisdom: "You better not fuck this up." Very motivating.

Having finished a painful first year transitioning from Catholic elementary school to even more mind-numbing public high school boredom, I was just days away from turning fifteen in the summer after freshman year when the water tower incident happened.

I remember it because I remember all of my failures with an overabundance of precision: every girl I turned down (I was so lacking in confidence at various points, I figured they were asking as a joke), treated poorly (there are one or two college girlfriends who rightly should still hate me) or disappointed (I have to guess at this list, but I'm sure there were several). I remember every person I angered or at least a long enough list that it seems like everyone. The Lutheran preacher I mistreated in the high school newspaper because I didn't do my job as a reporter properly. The disabled boyhood friends I only visited twice as an adult because I was too busy with my priorities, convincing myself I would see them more when I retired even though they had already far surpassed their life expectancy. People I fired to meet cost-savings targets without what I considered reasonable warning. Far too often, the person I disappointed most was myself, like when I rushed through a last paper while working on my master's degree. The poor result cost me a level of recognition I badly wanted because I was simply too tired or too lazy to put in the last bit of work. There's plenty more where these came from and, believe me, far worse.

If I remembered the highlights in my life as easily, the brief moments we should all live to savor, life would bring more pleasure. But my failures take a disproportionate amount of my memory capacity, even to this day. The only difference is I'm conscious of this now, and combat it by purposely thinking about reasons I have to be grateful. I've read that most people's memory helps them remember events with a more positive spin than how they actually occurred. I wish my mind did a better job of recasting my failures.

I remember the water tower incident, at least after the drug- and alcohol-induced unconsciousness passed, because it was the first time I recall seriously considering killing myself. I wasn't yet in the depths of depression, but I'd already started a steep downhill slide. From that height, my chances of immediate death if I jumped were high. It might not even hurt that bad since I was still at least ten hours away from sobriety, but death wasn't certain. With my luck, I'd leave myself paralyzed from the neck down and lose total control of my life—and death. I decided not to risk it. I was pretty sure I wanted to die, but clearly not yet certain. I'd already learned in football and too many childhood fights that I wasn't a big fan of physical pain. I didn't even know whether I hated pain more than I hated myself for hating pain.

So when I spotted what turned out to be Clarissa high up on a mountain north of Flagstaff in June of 2041, I thought again about that day, and many others, even as most of my focus turned to the awkward, gangly girl all alone and off trail, acting strangely not far below the tree line beneath Humphreys Peak.

As I walked close to her, my mind turned to questions: Is she the reason I'm alive? Is this one of the moments that makes the days, months and sometimes years of struggle worthwhile or will this encounter be another memory I struggle to shake?

Then I realized that the tall, thin-hipped body bent over a wood stick with ass pointed skyward belonged to a young girl, a teenager in all likelihood. Despite her baggy sweats, it was hard to turn my eyes away until it was clear that this rangy body belonged to a face so young. Even at a distance, something about her was captivating my attention. I didn't know why. When Clarissa looked toward me, though, I knew she needed me in her life. I couldn't let her down.

Already on that day, Clarissa had the makings of a beautiful woman. She might not have been a head-turner in high school terms, mind you, where beauty is defined as too much make-up, overly tight clothes, the right weight, perfect hair and other telling signs to a high school boy that a girl might gain portions of her self-worth or her own pleasure from satisfying his spear-motivated desires. Beautiful nonetheless. A pleasant, disarming face accented by high cheekbones. The rest of Clarissa was hidden under a baseball cap and overly loose clothing covered in a forest camouflage pattern.

Clarissa's body didn't appear to have filled in all of the parts boys seem to care about in tremendous disproportion to their long-term relationship satisfaction value. That, combined with being six feet tall at an age when she likely looked down at most classmates, meant Clarissa didn't get noticed the way girls who were perky, busty or smiling happily and frequently were noticed.

It was clear she must be overly thin from the taut appearance of her visible cheek. Still, she was clearly athletic enough to have hiked up here, so couldn't be devoid of physical strength. But anyone could see past Clarissa's effort to hide inside her own skin that she wasn't too many years away from catching more than her share of attention.

My seconds of evaluation as I ambled toward Clarissa reached conclusions about her solely based on physical appearance, even though this is the least important element of a soul's worth in this world.

Appearance was all I could see at this point. It was all I could initially judge.

When she looked again toward me as I drew near, I spotted more fear and pain in the eye I could see. That eye exposed a despair I fully recognized. Then I saw why she was bent over. It wasn't a wood stick wedged into the ground. It was a rifle. Her mouth remained over the barrel as her head turned partially so she could look at me with one eye.

Clarissa was reaching for the trigger.

3

Stopping Clarissa

THAT IMAGE, the one of Clarissa's mouth wrapped around the barrel of her rifle with her long arm stretching for the trigger, is one I can't wipe from my mind.

When alerted by my steps toward her, Clarissa peered at me with a single eye, almost greenish-hazel in color but otherwise devoid of detectable human connection. The detachment, the cold reticence in her eye, stood in stark contrast to tears rolling down the inside of her slightly over-sized nose only to turn sharply downward as gravity pulled each drop to the ground. As I looked at Clarissa, I saw emptiness, a drained spirit, an opacity I had only seen in others when I had been there for final minutes as humanity drained from their bodies. She looked past me even as I tried to get her attention.

I dreaded the next second with every ounce of my being, feeling my sternum and spine move opposite directions as my heart and lungs pounded between them. My guts churned as I moved as quickly forward as I could without startling her.

"I need your help, miss," I finally said to her, trying to buy time to think what I should do. I didn't particularly need help that day, a reasonably decent summer day even at these elevations. But I wanted her to know that I needed her to not pull the trigger. At that moment, I guess it helped me to know what it felt like to simply not care about living to see even the next second.

"What's your name, miss?" I asked, hoping she would pull her mouth off the barrel to respond. She looked at me out of that single eye for what seemed an eternity. A burst of cooler air passed through the nearby bristlecone pines, providing a momentary distraction. The sun continued to shine brightly on that early summer afternoon, giving the near-constant winds a measure of warmth to blow away. I tried to think as quickly as I could to figure out whatever I could to help this girl, but all I remember truly thinking was how long every second was taking and how petrified I was that I might be too late.

When she turned her eye away from me and looked back down, mouth still clenched around the barrel, I screamed out, "Oh God, no." I leapt toward her, unsure what I would do if I made it to her before the bullet reached her skull, but knowing I couldn't simply stand and watch.

Her right hand rose in the air, palm facing toward me telling me to stop. Her left hand still grasped the rifle barrel.

Then, reason for hope. Clarissa pulled her mouth off the rifle. She reached up with the sleeve of her thick sweatshirt to wipe her eyes, turning to look at me. The emptiness apparent just seconds ago was hidden behind a new mask: perhaps shame, perhaps fear, perhaps simply surprise.

"Can you help me?" I asked again.

She stared at me for several seconds. I could see life returning to her eyes, color to her pale, lightly freckled skin. I could also see her debating whether to return her mouth to the barrel and snap the trigger. She crossed her arms tightly in front of her and began biting her upper lip. Clarissa looked several times between the rifle and me as I tried to refocus her attention.

"I'm lost," I added as I continued my distraction efforts. I wasn't really lost, at least not any more than I was on any other day. Inside my backpack, I carried water, food, a puncture stick and a high-intensity tranquilizer gun I could use if I found myself being eyed as dinner. I also had my Lifelink mobile device, the all-in-one computer, identification, and payment device that I struggled to learn in my old age. The device has a great global positioning system and hike-mapping program that could tell me where I was and the most efficient way to get wherever I was going. Just about fifteen hundred feet down from the peak of the highest mountain in Arizona, I could also simply look around and have a good sense of where I was as I had done for years hiking throughout the United States, with particular fondness for the Southwest.

I have long known it was odd that a man in his seventies would hike on his own, but no one in my immediate family thought much of the outdoors. "If wanting to sleep in a bed makes me a princess, you can queen me," my wife had told me soon after we married when I neglected to make motel reservations during a weekend hike in West Virginia's Appalachian Mountains in the midst of fall color season.

In a strange way, I also enjoyed hiking completely alone. Perhaps the ability to enjoy time alone is one of the gifts of introversion, a stark contrast to the panic I frequently felt and consciously struggled to control when placed in front of large groups or even new people over the years. Gaining that ability to be comfortable alone had been a survival mechanism at one point in my life. Once acquired, I was reluctant to part from the comfort if offered me.

None of it mattered at that moment. Clarissa needed to know that I needed her.

"I'm Mike," I said, extending my hand to shake hers and trying to give her reason to be calm. "I hiked way too far today and need help getting back to safety. Can you help me? Please."

Clarissa's chest dropped. Her shoulders sagged. She dropped her head and looked back at the ground. Even over the gusts at these oxygen-deprived heights, I could hear her take several deep breaths.

"I'm Clarissa," she finally responded with no hint of emotion in her voice.

"Nice to meet you Clarissa. I'm so glad I found you. I don't know what I would have done if I was stuck here overnight. I'm clearly not prepared to camp over-night."

"Well. It is what it is. I guess I can help you . . . I guess."

"Thank you. I'll be eternally grateful," I replied. "Clarissa, right?"

"Yeah, Clarissa. Clarissa Co . . . ," she started to say. "Clarissa."

"Do you mind heading down now, Clarissa?" I asked, trying to keep her moving and fixated on something other than what she clearly came here to do.

"No, that's fine, I guess," she told me. "We may as well get going."

Clarissa looked at me and I looked at her. I wasn't quite sure whether what I saw in her eyes was annoyance, relief or pain, but at least I could see emotion. I looked around for her backpack. She didn't have one. Her only company was this odd-looking rifle.

"Would you like some water?" I asked. I was relieved when she took my canteen. There's no reason to drink water if you aren't at least contemplating sticking around for the rest of the day.

"How fast can you move, Grandpa, I mean mister, uhhh, Mike?" Clarissa finally asked.

"Grandpa?" I responded, feigning indignity. "I'll beg you to slow down if I can't keep up, but otherwise don't worry about me."

In those moments, my mind raced with questions I wanted to ask, statements I wanted to make, wisdom I needed to share. All in due time, I thought. All in due time.

We began the hike down. Clarissa was kind. I have no doubt she would have moved at a much faster pace on her own, but then, it was also clear to me that she came here with no intention of descending.

Weaving around pines, spruces and firs that dominated the environment as we moved down from the tree line, it wasn't long before the tree clusters were too thick to maintain a clear visual of our direction. On my own, I would have pulled out my Lifelink and used it to guide me out or at least back to the trail. But I couldn't let Clarissa know I didn't need her. She needed to know she had a purpose even if all I could offer her today was a temporary goal.

I watched intently as Clarissa took the rifle I had initially confused for a wood hiking stick and turned it into exactly that. "That's pretty cool. I never saw anything like that before," I said, trying my best to make conversation. "How does it work?"

Then I saw it: a hint of a smile. Clearly, she wasn't ready for joy or happiness, but perhaps I could help her gain a measure of calm? What could possibly be so awful to stick her mouth on that barrel?

"My dad made it. It works as a rifle, a spear or a club, if I need it," she responded in a very soft, nearly monotonous tone I had to strain to hear. "You never know what you're going to run into in the wild. I like that it just looks like a normal hiking stick. That way, when I run into other people while I'm hiking, they don't freak out."

"I can see that," I responded, racing my next thought through potential reactions before letting it out. "I have to tell you, that rifle mode freaked me out so I'm so happy you put it away."

I wanted to see if I could make a connection, so I asked Clarissa if we could take a rest on a downed tree for a few minutes.

"I would have asked what you were doing back there," I said to her before we reached a place to sit. "But I'm pretty sure I know. I don't know why you're so unhappy. I don't know what made you despondent and so empty you can't see a better choice . . ."

"Do you want my fucking help or not?" she reacted in clear rage. Damn it. I pushed too hard, too soon. I began to panic that I might lose her attention. But then, several seconds later, she spoke again, far more softly. "I'm sorry, I didn't need to barf at you."

"Barf?" I asked. "I know I'm old, but I don't see any vomit."

"You know. Swearing. Cursing. Whatever old people call it," Clarissa blurted.

I breathed with a bit of a sigh. She thought about my feelings enough to apologize. That's great, but I needed to figure out what was going on in her head.

We had already put what seemed like one thousand feet of elevation between where I spotted Clarissa and where we stood when a good spot to sit opened in front of us. For those who don't hike regularly, a thousand-foot descent feels at least like walking down one hundred flights of stairs. It's certainly much easier than climbing up, and I could move down much faster than I could go up when the combination of stressful work and tightening oxygen deprivation really stressed every bit of my heart and lungs.

I love this part of any hike. Every muscle in my body is already aching, but there's a sense of accomplishment that comes from having reached a goal. Getting to the top of a peak on a hard but doable path like Humphreys trail might not seem like an extraordinary goal, but it sure beats having a successful bowel movement as a day's accomplishment. Most days, I'm happy to have done something that can proudly fill ninety seconds of conversation with a family member. I can talk about a hike like this for almost as long as it takes me to finish the hike. Whether anyone will sit and listen that long is another matter. Reaching goals gives me the moments of satisfaction that make the difficulties of day-to-day life worth enduring. Being outdoors and being mobile are two of my greatest pleasures in life. At that moment, I was fortunate to still have both.

Everything in sight was a spectacle. It's funny how different we are as people. Five minutes into looking at even the grandest natural scenery, my wife would be bored and ready to escape before any bugs moved within range. I could sit writing or reading in a single spot in the woods all day and never run out of wonder. At that point, there was enough space between the trees that the light blue noon sky radiated above, colored only by white cloud wisps and speckled by the occasional bird searching for food. The barren views of alpine tundra and moon-like rock near the summit of Humphreys Peak were distant memory here, as were the bristlecone pines at tree line. We sat in a lush evergreen forest, listening to woodpeckers providing a high-intensity drumbeat with a backing track of whistling winds, birds chirping and ground being displaced by the occasional scampering forest animal.

"What do you see here?" I asked Clarissa as we took seats on long dead tree trunks where we could face each other.

"A bunch of trees. Some dirt. Some rocks," she responded in monotone voice. "Why?"

"I grew up camping as a kid, so I've always loved the space and beauty of nature. It's where I come to find peace. So I see branches twisted into odd shapes, and the blues in the sky and greens on the trees, but what I really see is perspective."

"Perspective?" she asked.

"Perspective," I replied. "Let me ask you some questions. How would you describe that Douglas fir over there?" I asked, pointing to a particular tree.

"Beautiful I guess."

"How about those bristlecone pines where we first met, the ones with more trunk and limb than needles?"

"Yeah, I'm not sure about beautiful, but they're interesting," she responded, a bit of exasperation clear in her voice.

"How about all those ponderosa pines?" I asked, pointing to a broad patch nearby.

"Sure, clean, strong, whatever."

"How about the . . ." I started to ask before Clarissa interrupted.

"Yeah, I don't really know what everything is called here, but I'll give you that everything in nature is either beautiful or interesting or certainly, you know, I guess useful," she acknowledged.

"It all has a purpose, but it's all different. Right?" I said as more of a statement than a question. "And the interesting part is that the environment, the world, needs all of this variety to survive and prosper. It's all interconnected. We're all interconnected. We all need each other, even if we don't always know why at any given moment. That's the perspective I'm reminded of when I'm out hiking."

"I don't want to talk about this any more," she said, sweatpants billowing in the wind around her long, thin legs as she moved again. "Come on. If you want my help."

"Clarissa. I not only want your help. I need your help," I said, trying to ignore the creaks and cracks as I began following. It takes several minutes for my muscles to warm up and move at a decent pace, so I had to watch my step and keep an eye on where Clarissa was going at the same time.

"But I also know what it feels like to want the pain to end. Like you were doing up there," I yelled out in much louder voice.

Clarissa stopped, looking around to see if anyone heard me, then turned toward me with her eyes pointing down to the dirt. Her face turned red, whether from anger or embarrassment I couldn't yet determine. Clearly, she had to be sure I could never really understand. In some ways she would be right. Do we ever really know what it feels like to be another person? Of course not, and certainly not after just knowing someone for perhaps an hour, the length of time I had then known Clarissa.

"How could you possibly know what I feel like?" she asked, stammering through the last few words. Her cheeks began to tremor, as the dormant volcano beneath this peak once did. Tears flowed out of Clarissa as she sat back down on a low, rounded rock and buried her head into her arms.

I walked over and gently touched her shoulders, not wanting to frighten her, but not wanting her to feel physically alone as she clearly already must feel. At that moment I remembered the worst of my teenage pain, when I went out of my way to avoid even a hug from my mother because it reminded me how empty I felt.

"Did you really know what I was trying to do?" Clarissa finally asked, lifting her head slightly as she spoke, but not enough that I could see her face. Her fists wedged up tightly against her thighs.

"I knew, and I knew I couldn't let you make a mistake I almost made myself, probably at about the age you are now," I said.

"Really?"

"Why don't we walk slowly so I can tell you about being a fifteen-year-old boy, sitting on the train tracks in my hometown in the middle of the night, twisting a knife I stole from work right under my rib cage, trying to decide whether to plunge it in," I said, staring intently at Clarissa.

"Really?"

"Really. But before I tell you my story, I want to hear about you. Tell me what you were thinking up there," I said, turning on a video recorder built into my glasses and handing her a microphone clip to clasp on her bottom lip. "I won't show this to anyone without your permission."

{ 4 }

Meeting Mike

CLARISSA TOOK THE LIP CLIP and pulled her cap down to cover her eyes. The camera didn't really capture much of Clarissa as we walked, since the lens is built into my glasses and I mainly focused on where I would take my next step. It took some time to talk Clarissa into recording what she was thinking, but I thought it might be helpful to her to hear herself talk about how she felt. At least I was hoping it would help. At the very least, it would buy me time to think about what to do. The longer I could separate her from that moment of desperation the better.

Already Clarissa was more than a human form to me. She was real: a person with feelings, not an abstract number or concept. As evergreens thinned at points through our walk, the reddish tint of the back of her rolled-up hair would reflect the sun, adding to the natural colors around. She walked in front of me or near my side most of the time, so I saw her face only intermittently.

Finally, Clarissa agreed to talk if I would agree to just shut up so she could think and if I would message the recording to her when I was done. I couldn't really hear as much of what she said as I would have liked at the time, but I picked up the gist of what she was saying.

"So, uhmm. Hi. Uhh. I don't know if I want to do this. Well, what could it hurt, really?"

At this point, Clarissa stopped to make sure I wouldn't share anything she said with anyone. I promised I wouldn't without her approval.

"What am I thinking? I'm thinking that I'm angry. I'm angry at you for showing up, angry at me for being a wimp and angry at the world for being cruel to me. I was finally ready to just end it when you interfered with my moment. I'd finished final preparations— converting my hiking stick into rifle mode. In a way, I felt bad that I was using the stick because my dad made it for us to defend ourselves in the wild without scaring other hikers and he'd probably be mad than I used it to kill myself but it was the only gun I could get besides the tranquilizer gun without him wondering what I was doing.

"Before you showed up, I wrote a note and shoved it into my pants in case my body was discovered before the animals found me and fully turned my body into a scat assortment. I guess I'll give it to you, because that's what I was thinking," Clarissa said as she reached down inside her sweats, pulled out the note and handed it to me.

"I mean, it's embarrassing and it's pretty bad writing, I know, but it's not like I write anything out ever without a computer to fix it all up and it's not like I was worried about my paper being graded.

"But then, when you came up on me, I was taking one last look around, kind of looking down at the city. Flagstaff doesn't look so bad from up here. It's just down there that I don't belong. I had to escape. I'd thought about just running away or disappearing into the woods and living on my own because that seems to be the only time I'm happy anymore. But I'm pretty sure I'd end up miserable on my own or tied up in some creep's cabin even more abused and with no way to just die.

"But I needed to get away for good. Doing this, ending it, felt like the best way to go. I mean, people just die or get hurt if they're around me anyway, so why not get it over with and keep that from happening to more people?"

Clarissa stopped talking for a moment and started to pull off the lip clip microphone to hand back to me. I hadn't come up with any good ideas on what to do next so I asked her to tell me about something she finds painful. It took a bit of doing, but she took the clip back, put it on her bottom lip, walked closer to me, and began talking again.

"I've been hurting for as long as I can remember, but things seemed to start getting worse around sixth grade," Clarissa said in the recording. "I grew a lot that year and got way taller than everyone else in my classes. I couldn't control my body. Everyone made fun of me all the time. I was giraffe, snake, skeleton, and always like I didn't belong and no one wanted me around. I just wanted to curl up in a corner and hide. I mean, I had friends, right. But, not many friends and I was always like the last one of the group. I always felt better around older people.

"Then, when I got my . . . uhhmmm . . . period, right in the middle of freakin' gym class. Oh, this is embarrassing to talk about, but what the hell. It's not like you're gonna make fun of me, are you Mike?" Clarissa said, turning to look at me. "I mean, you wouldn't do that, I don't think."

I shook my head to assure her that I would not.

"I was hoping I was just sweating until a little blood started seeping through my shorts. Billy Kunzler noticed before I did. It could have been almost anyone else without being so miserable but it had to be Billy.

"'Hey, everybody,' Billy yelled out, pointing at my shorts. 'Looks like Clarissa wants to play Red Rover. Red Rover, Red Rover, come on over.'

"What an asshole. He could have just come up to me and told me I was bleeding. That would have been humiliating enough. But, no. He has to tell the whole class and everyone laughs at me. He started telling all the boys that my period was the sign I wanted to do him, like he even knew what that meant. What an idiot. I wish I could have gotten over it or forgotten it but too many people keep reminding me. They think it's just hilarious.

"I mean, how would you feel if everywhere you walk, people just start laughing at you? That was the start of open season on Clarissa and it's continued ever since," Clarissa added, ingrained pain apparent from her expressions.

I was shaking my head in sympathy with her as she finished. "You know, that's pretty remarkable," I said.

"What's remarkable?"

"That you have the confidence to talk about painful experiences like that," I replied.

"You think this is confidence?"

"Well, it seems that way," I noted.

"It's not confidence. It's more like just wanting someone to know how I feel and you're here and you can't ruin my life any more than it's already ruined," Clarissa said.

"Well, it still seems brave to me," I told her, then asked her to continue telling me about why she thinks she has become so unhappy.

"Look, I tried my best to hide. But after four years of hiding I just can't take it anymore. This year has been even worse," Clarissa continued.

"First, my Grandpa gets killed. We lived with him, so he was around all the time and he seemed like the only one who had any time for me anymore. Mom and Dad were always so busy at work and my sisters think I'm a spoiled brat tomboy not worthy of their time. Then the police say Grandpa was threatening people with his rifle and calling them racist names and they attacked him and knocked him over and he died. So they started telling everyone that our whole family was racist and the few girls who were nice to me decided when I got back that they wouldn't be my friends anymore. So I have no one to talk to and I'm alone all the time. I can't wait for every day to end and I dread every damn morning. You know, it pisses me off when I wake up and find out I'm still here."

I did my best to back off and keep Clarissa from remembering I was there. She was on a roll, starting to open up and I didn't want to interfere. As much as I wanted to hear what she was saying as she spoke, I figured I'd listen to it later rather than get so close that she might clam up.

"Right after that happened with Grandpa, I met this new friend, Sarah. She's an older woman, really successful. One of the fiercest warriors in the country, ex-Navy Seal, and a really vibing person, the kind anyone would think was cool to hang out with. Well, I met her anyway at this survival camp place my family went to and she went out and searched and found me when I got lost. I could tell she actually cared about me. For a few days, I thought that maybe someone important did notice I existed and made me feel like I could do something with my life and really, actually cared about me without needing to be forced to pretend to care. She came out to where I was camped at later and we just sat there staring off at a lake and talking about life and she was really interesting and I felt like for the first time in years maybe my life didn't have to suck. Imagine that. Somebody actually gave a damn about me. I wasn't Camel Toe Clarissa or Clarissa Cuntman or Creepy Clarissa or any of the things Billy and his friends call me. I was just Clarissa. The next day after that, she's gone and she's dead. I mean, how cruel is that? I guess I'm just a horrible jinx on everyone.

"I've tried since then to not feel like shit, but nothing I do has worked. I feel like I'm walking around with a five-hundred-pound weight on my back, making everything I do painful and then smothering me if I ever start moving and feel like I'm making progress. I keep thinking about dropping out and running away and just starting somewhere new, but how do I know it wouldn't be just as bad or worse."

Clarissa paused for a bit. She looked at me and I just looked back at her, wanting to encourage her to continue. After what seemed an eternity when I listened to it later, but was really only a minute, she started talking again.

"I used to really love coming up here in the mountains, hiking on my own to get away," she added. "At least no one was nasty to me up here and I felt like I was doing something worth remembering. But since I came back from the Utah camp when Grandpa and Sarah were killed, I haven't even felt the energy to go hiking or walking or anything anymore. I've always been too skinny, but now I don't even have any muscle left and I never feel like eating and I'm just so gross and disgusting."

Clarissa was so far from me at this point, I wasn't even getting pieces of what she was saying until I listened later.

"So, what am I thinking? Actually, I'm still thinking I should've just pulled the trigger. From the moment I took my mouth off the rifle, I couldn't get you to shut up until you gave me the mike clip. I mean, seriously, I wondered if you were ever gonna just shut up and leave me alone. I was trying to think and you're spitting out questions like I just burned the house down.

"Can you help me? What do you think of the pretty tree? How's that rifle made? Can I hold it for you? What do you think I am, some moron who's gonna give my gun to a creepy old guy I've known for five minutes? What are you gonna do, threaten to shoot me if I don't follow your orders? Go ahead and kill me anyway. Can't you see that was the plan?" Clarissa was on a roll, talking so fast I had to replay parts of her message to be sure I heard them properly.

"I feel totally jinxed. I can't even kill myself right. I'm such a pathetic, miserable loser. I can't even kill myself with my mouth already on the barrel of the rifle and my finger pretty much on the trigger.

"I mean, am I really that awful of a person? I don't hurt people. I can't believe I'm just plain stupid but maybe I am. I know I'm ugly. I've had enough boys and girls tell me that I just know. If I would have just pulled the trigger, you could've stopped listening to this and got on with your happy life and not heard me babbling.

"I guess what I really want to know is why does everyone else get to be happy and I have to feel like shit all the time? I mean I was actually looking forward to death, that's how bad I felt."

After another pause in which all I heard was the soft rustling of her steps in piles of pine needles, Clarissa continued.

"Do you know, Mike, how pissed I was when you pretended that you knew how I felt and you're telling me that I'm desperate or depressed or something. How could you possibly know how I feel? Do your hormones rage every month? No one's ever started Red Rover games in the middle of math class just to ridicule you. I shoulda walked away as soon as I got you to the path, but I figured you weren't gonna leave me alone.

"Then you start telling me you were gonna kill yourself when you were my age. At first, I decided this had to be a crock of crap. I've heard better lies out of Billy when he was trying to shove his hands down my pants," Clarissa added, before switching to talk in a deep, annoying boy voice. "'I always loved you, Clarissa. That's why I made fun of you all the time. I wanted you to notice me.' What a load of shit. He woulda stuck his hands down my pants and then ran around telling all his friends to smell his finger. Total despicable jerk. I want a boy who's proud to be with me, not someone to just use me or make me a joke for his friends. Ugghhh."

Clarissa came closer to me at this point.

"I don't want anyone to hear this because they'd probably just hate me more. I'm really not a mean person. You don't hate me now, do you?" Clarissa asked, turning to look directly in my eyes.

"Of course not," I replied. "Of course not."

She asked me to turn off the recording, send it to her and then delete it. I complied with her first two requests.

{ 5 }

Going Down

W E WALKED, SLOWLY AND SIDE-BY-SIDE when we fit on the path down. When the path narrowed, or a few hikers passed us on their way up for an overnight stay, I would try to get in front so I could still hear Clarissa speak in her soft, unsure, clearly reluctant voice. She took time to gather her thoughts frequently; unsurprising, given that few fully understand what drives their desperation when they get to the point they no longer want to live.

"I just can't take it anymore," Clarissa began, pausing, stopping and looking at me. "You're not going to tell anyone this, are you?" she asked.

"I'll tell you what, Clarissa," I responded. "If you don't tell anyone about me, I won't tell anyone about you." I realized as I finished saying this that I was lying so I added, "I need to be honest. I won't tell anyone you don't want me to tell as long as I can know you're getting help and going to be okay. Otherwise, I can't just let you hurt yourself."

"You can't tell anyone. Promise me. Promise me or I'm done talking," she said more energetically than her typical soft, barely discernible voice.

"Okay, okay. I promise, but why is what others think so important to you?" I asked, flashing my hands upward and out.

"I don't want anyone to think I'm crazy. The only thing I've ever thought I could be happy at is being in the military. Do you think the Navy Seals take nut jobs?" Clarissa asked.

"I don't know, but I'm certain they don't take corpses," I replied, realizing that my attempt at humor was off the mark only after the statement left my lips. I hadn't used my brain as a filter. "Sorry, I don't mean to be glib about this."

"I guess you're at least technically right," she replied, gently letting me off the hook. "If my government health record shows mental illness, I'm automatically excluded from Special Forces eligibility. And I know my dad or the government will take away my guns."

I hadn't seen any of this coming and was immediately struck that I needed someone who knows what they are doing to talk with this girl. I was in way over my head.

I thought about leaving it alone, but how could I? I couldn't just ignore that what she was thinking on her own wasn't leading her to a good place. Even though I was no expert at how to deal with her specific issues, I wasn't about to stop trying with Clarissa until I could at least ensure there was someone in her life capable of helping.

"So, let me get this straight. The only career you think will make you happy requires that you have a clean mental health record. You're depressed enough to stick a rifle into your mouth, but you're so worried about people finding out that you're depressed that you won't get help. And, with no hope of help without talking to someone, you'll probably end up back at the tree line," I said, or maybe I just thought this, but I'm pretty sure I said most of it out loud again without sifting the thoughts through a clearly overwhelmed mind.

I grabbed Clarissa from the front by her shoulders and looked into her eyes. She backed her face away.

At first, I thought Clarissa was either worried I was getting creepy or just uncomfortable that a stranger had invaded her space. There was a third possibility. Human connection is tough for someone who feels alone and desperate, whose depression has deteriorated to suicidal thoughts or actions. During those many months when I cycled in and out of my worst depression as a teen, I did my best to avoid getting or staying close to anyone. Connection meant I might leave something meaningful behind.

"I won't tell anyone, but you have to promise to keep talking to me, at least until I can help you understand something that took me many years to understand," I said as I fixated on her.

Clarissa pulled back further from my hands.

Seconds later, a lightning bolt struck just a few hundred feet away, slicing deeply through a nearby pine and shearing it down the middle. The top portion of the tree crashed to the ground with a loud thud that sent dozens of nearby birds streaming from their perches. In the distance, I spotted a small black bear running for cover. I warned Clarissa to look out. We searched in a circle to make sure we weren't going to be caught between the cub and its mother.

Clarissa grabbed her wood hiking stick and flipped open a panel I hadn't noticed before. She keyed in a three-digit code and a long knife shot out the end of the stick to turn it into a spear. I scrambled for the tranquilizer gun in my backpack.

"It's lightning out here. You don't want to be holding onto metal," I barked.

"There's also something like one hundred thousand trees that are one hundred feet tall," Clarissa responded. "I'm more worried about the bear's mother.

Besides, we need to find shelter. It looks like we're about to be dumped on."

At least for the moment, Clarissa was willing to fight to prevent herself from suffering a prolonged, excruciatingly painful death.

I followed Clarissa, who clearly had come hiking on Humphreys trail many more times than my several hikes over the decades and was no longer worried about whether I could keep pace. We crossed off the path with our sight obscured by ever-thickening forest. Though she is an inch taller than I was at my tallest, and is probably two or three inches taller than I am now, Clarissa had no problem ducking under branches. Her long legs made it easy for her to step over boulders and tree trunks while hardly breaking stride. I struggled mightily to keep up before being jolted by a noise from my backpack.

My heart monitor alarm was blaring, letting me know I had surpassed my maximum heart rate for safe exercise. We had moved so quickly, I don't recall even hearing the quick beep that should have warned me I was approaching my maximum heart rate.

"What's that?" Clarissa yelled back.

"Nothing to worry about," I responded, not wanting to pull out my Lifelink and give away that I had access to trail mapping applications. "Just a heart monitor alert telling me to slow down."

"Okay, we're almost there," she yelled back as rain began to pelt us both.

Almost where, I wondered? I couldn't see anything through the rain except trees, rocks and dirt. I was reaching full annoyance with pine needles scraping exposed skin on my hands, face and neck. It wouldn't take long for those scrapes to turn into unsightly collections of cuts and bruises. The rain at least is washing the dirt away, but I knew I was going to be cold.

Then, there it was.

"My little cave," Clarissa announced from under a rock overhang that wasn't really a cave, stretching her left hand like a game show hostess or flight attendant giving safety instructions. "Welcome to my summer hideaway."

I hadn't smiled that much all day, but the broad smile that came over my face was part relief and part joy that this young girl who seemed a lost soul just hours earlier was showing small signs of life.

"I can't begin to tell you how thrilled I am to not be hiking back in the rain. I thought storm season here didn't start until later in the summer."

The view from the top of Humphreys Peak is spectacular and varied, making it a fairly popular hiking destination. On a clear day, as I had seen earlier in late morning, a part of the Grand Canyon captures the initial visual attention of most hikers. The peak itself is barren, with almost all of its snowcap having melted to refresh surrounding water supplies. Coated with pebbles, rocks and boulders of varying sizes, the peak could just as easily have been a lunar landing spot if not for the spectacular scenery in the distance.

I left that morning at nearly dawn for the day's hike. I hadn't been able to convince anyone to accompany me on this hiking trip. My wife was never an outdoorsy type, something I first learned during our honeymoon. "You know all that canoeing and hiking and picnicking stuff we did when we were dating?" she said to me while I consumed a second entrée at an all-inclusive resort in Montego Bay, Jamaica. "Yeah, I don't do that." She denies having said this so clearly, and has accompanied me on a few short hikes over the years, but the outdoors are not her thing, unless we're talking sand and sun.

The view from Humphreys Peak—the real one after having been tricked three times earlier into thinking I was at the peak—had been worth all the hard work to get there that morning. I rested for thirty minutes in the aggressive winds at the peak to enjoy viewing a bit of the Grand Canyon, parts of Flagstaff that are only seven or eight miles away, and a bunch of steep white hills that looked every bit like natural monuments set up for the enjoyment of Humphreys Peak hikers.

Clarissa was camping with her father and sisters years earlier when she found this spot. The overhang itself isn't that far from the trail, but few of the thousands who hike the trails ever go this direction. It is quiet. Clarissa could truly be herself here without worrying about anyone else. The spot near the tree line where I had first noticed her was another of Clarissa's favorite locations on the mountain to be alone.

Finally after a bit of silence and doing my best to dry off, Clarissa and I sat against the back of the mountain rock. The wind was blowing enough that rain, which never would have touched us if it came straight down, was splashing up on our tucked-in feet.

"Can I tell you something?" Clarissa asked after some time.

"Of course."

"I thought you were someone else when I stopped trying to pull the trigger," she noted.

"Someone else?" I asked.

She looked at the ground. "I thought you were my grandpa."

"Why would you think that?"

"I don't know. You don't even look that much like him now. But when I looked at you at first, you did," Clarissa said, her face reverting to sullen tension and her arms again crossed tightly in front of her.

"So, if you could tell I wasn't your grandpa right away, were you really going to pull the trigger?" I asked.

"I was, if I coulda figured out how to get my fingerprint accepted. My dad put a fingerprint ID pad on his weapons so only those of us trained in the family can shoot the rifles. I guess he never considered how the fingerprint would work if the barrel was pointed at us," she suggested.

"Or perhaps, he did," I replied. I gave her a few seconds to consider that her father's wisdom in designing the weapon may have helped save his daughter's life. The rain outside intensified, deeply soaking the area.

"Do you believe that events in our lives have reasons or value, Clarissa, even if we can't possibly fathom what those reasons might be at the time?" I questioned.

"I don't know," she responded before asking where I was from. "Okay, Mike from Illinois, what reasons are you talking about?" she said in prompting the conversation to continue.

"Reasons, like me taking a wrong turn off the trail and ending up standing near you, or like you looking at me and seeing your grandpa at exactly the time you needed to see your grandpa. I almost get the feeling that he sent me to you. I could have been on any of thousands of trails, or not had things happen that made me want to be hiking this week, this day. If any of this changed, you wouldn't have seen him when you looked up. Doesn't that just seem strange to you?"

"I guess," Clarissa replied. "But if he hadn't been killed, maybe I wouldn't be quite as angry. He would have helped me. He would've at least cared." She dropped her head and shook it back and forth. She was trying to reject this concept of fate, but I don't think she could quite convince herself it was wrong. "I can't believe God, if there even is a God, murdered my grandpa so you could see me today. That just doesn't make any sense. It just doesn't seem fair."

"It does sound a bit far-fetched when you think about it," I responded. "But then I think about all that had to have happened for me to meet you. I think about what made me decide not to plunge that knife through my heart so many years ago. Was meeting you one of the reasons I was meant to stay alive? And, if there is a God, did he send me to you, or did he send you here to save me?"

"Why would I need to save you?" Clarissa asked, looking more puzzled than she had all afternoon.

"That's a good question," I replied. "We can talk about that later."

We sat in silence for a while. I was trying to figure out what to say next. Clarissa stared at the rain.

"Do you really believe in fate?" Clarissa finally asked after perhaps ten minutes of silence.

"I don't know if I would call what I believe in 'fate,'" I replied, making visual quote marks as I spoke. "At least not in the way most people talk about fate. But I do think each of us has a purpose, an intrinsic worth and beauty that we don't always see in ourselves. I mean, think about it. Does a tree see its own value and worth when a woodpecker is burrowing into it or a bird is crapping on it and a squirrel is clawing at its bark? I can't imagine it would enjoy those experiences if it had human emotion. Who likes to be pecked at, crapped on or clawed at? No one I know. But to someone standing in front of the tree, they see majesty or beauty or strength or purpose, or maybe some combination of all those attributes. If that tree isn't there, it's not getting dumped on or clawed, but it's also not there to provide shade or produce food or hold the soil together to prevent erosion or whatever that tree does."

"You're losing me," Clarissa said, shaking her head.

"I'm sorry. Let me try again," I offered, pausing to gather my thoughts. "What I'm saying is that it's not so much that I believe our fate is determined and there's nothing we can do to affect it, because I don't believe that at all. We all have choices we make in our lives that affect our direction. I know that when I eat too much, I'm going to gain weight. When I get fat, my sleep apnea gets worse and when my apnea gets worse,

I'm going to be too tired to hike and gain more weight, et cetera. But I don't believe I'm fated to eat every time or everything I think about eating. It's a choice. Just one I struggle with all the time."

"My grandpa used to talk like you," Clarissa interjected, shaking her head as she spoke.

"So fate isn't that we can't control aspects of our lives," I continued after making sure Clarissa had said all she wanted to say. "Fate is that we're presented with people and moments in life and have decisions to make on how to respond to them," I added. "And at various points in my life, I've felt like particular moments are why I endured what I've endured. Like now. There are too many variables that had to come together for me to meet you when and where I did. Or like when I was in college, I wrote a column for *The Daily Illini* newspaper about my experience in high school with depression and suicidal thoughts."

"You told people about feeling like this?" Clarissa asked with a clear expression of surprise that included elevated eyebrows.

"I did, but really only in very select circumstances. I certainly didn't say anything in high school. I just wasn't that brave. And I only wrote about it my senior year in college, after I had accomplished what I could there and was ready to graduate. I hid it from most people for most of my life, until I finally reached a point where I could feel comfortable in my own skin and start talking about it more openly."

"When was that?" Clarissa asked. I sat and thought for a long time, trying to place the age when I thought sharing my history was more important than protecting my ego.

"God, I had to be close to fifty. I mean, I had told a few people before then, but always people I thought needed to know they weren't alone in how they felt. But, nothing broader than that," I noted.

"Do you remember what you wrote in college?" Clarissa asked, promisingly making full eye contact.

"Let's see if I can find it," I responded, pulling out my Lifelink mobile device, the combination computer, communicator, credit system that had long been an essential part of everyday life. Normally kept in sealed, code-protected inside shirt pockets, I had put mine into a coded backpack pocket for this hike.

As I opened it and began to search for old columns I had written in the pre-internet age, Clarissa realized I had everything I needed to get back down from the mountain on my own. I had forgotten that I didn't want her to know I had my Lifelink with me.

"You told me you needed me," Clarissa yelled, anger and then sadness growing with each word. Her clenched fists wedged inside her thighs, as if they would burst toward me if she didn't hold them there.

"With your Lifelink, you could get anywhere you want to go without me. Why didn't you just leave me up there to kill myself? I could have been done with this already."

I looked at her for several seconds, seeing pain take over her expression, not sure what I could possibly say. I couldn't come up with any thoughtful words but fortunately found the article I was looking for and clicked it up to display as I folded out the paper-thin device into full-screen mode.

"Read this," I finally said. "I think this will tell you why."

Clarissa took my Lifelink and began to scroll through the page views displayed from the opinion pages of *The Daily Illini* on May 7, 1986.

"After one particularly bad issue and a series of miserable events, my thoughts turned from whether to kill myself to how I would do it," I wrote in a column in which I bemoaned the apparent suicide of a university student who had jumped from his tenth floor window. "After a particularly bad day . . . I brought a knife along for company on my walk home. After walking four blocks, I sat down on an abandoned section of the railroad tracks that went through town and started smoking the marijuana that had become my hidden crutch. I loosened up with my joint, then put the tip of the blade up to my abdomen. Did I really want to do this? I was sick of everyone telling me how worthless I was. I had no talent for anything. No one would give a damn in any case. I wondered if anyone would even notice.

"But when it came down to it, I couldn't do it. Rather, I wouldn't do it. I didn't want to die. It was just that I didn't want to have to deal with feeling worthless all of the time. I couldn't afford to take everything personally. I had to walk away as much as possible from the people and things that had been messing up my life. At the same time, I had to work harder at improving some of my faults. And if things got worse, I promised to walk away from the place, not my life."

Clarissa stopped reading at this point, leaned over to put her head against my shoulder and began crying. My shirt had been drying out, but now my sleeve was being soaked all over again. I reached around to hold her, putting my left hand on the back of her head. It wasn't long before I blubbered a bit in sympathy as well. The rain wasn't a concern anymore. I was caught up in the raw and often painful emotion that comes from real human connection. While crying, I felt another bit of my lifelong self-worth trepidation and still too-frequent self-loathing seeping away. There's something life affirming about having a sense of purpose, particularly if that purpose is helping someone stave off death.

Several minutes later, Clarissa likely realized how long we had been holding each other and remembered a lifetime of admonitions about strangers. She pulled away, sat back up, then put her hand back on my shoulder and asked what I considered a truly insightful question.

"Do you ever regret not doing it?" she asked. "I mean, not, just, I guess, just killing yourself and getting rid of the pain."

"Well, if the question is do I ever get depressed, or feel bad, or wish I hadn't been around to experience some horrible event or do something stupid myself, then the answer is that life brings bad days and sometimes those bad days string together for a very, very long time. But I can't imagine never having played with or coached my kids, never enjoying the best of moments with my wife, never feeling the satisfaction of achievements, even missing moments like talking with you now and other real connections with real people. If I knew when I was your age all the good I would miss out on, even knowing all the struggle, pain and hard work that comes with it, I never would have wanted to kill myself."

I looked at Clarissa to make sure she understood. "Why don't you read the rest of the article," I said, "if you're interested?"

She turned the display screen back toward her eyes.

"I quit smoking pot and lowered my expectations on what I needed to accomplish in life. I decided to give it another week. Things couldn't stay that bad, I hoped. I wasn't happy at the end of the week, but things weren't so bad that the thought of killing myself was a constant battle. Another week passed. Then something funny happened. Someone complimented me," the article said.

"What do you mean about lowered your expectations?" Clarissa asked.

"I mean, I needed to stop living a life of envy," I responded.

"What?" she asked. "What does that mean?"

"I needed to stop wanting to live someone else's life. I had to stop caring that other people were better looking, better athletes, funnier, more sociable. I had to worry about being the best Mike that I could be," I told her, between taking sips from my canteen and passing it to Clarissa so she could drink as well. "You know all those people who tell you that you can achieve anything you want in life if you just work hard enough?"

"Yeah, my dad tells me that," Clarissa replied.

"Oh, well, no offense to him, but he's missing some key caveats. You know what caveats are, right?"

"I'm not stupid," she exclaimed, clearly annoyed.

"Sorry, I get told that I use words sometimes that real people don't use."

Clarissa nodded that she might agree with that statement. "So, what's the caveat?"

"You can accomplish anything you want in life, but only if you have the core basic talent, if you are both tenacious in pursuing your goal and patient in waiting for it to happen, and if you get a little bit of luck from finding so many places and times to display your talent that eventually you find yourself in the right time and place. Even then, your success might not look at all like you envisioned or happen as fast as you desired, but you wake up one day and say to yourself, I actually feel good about myself."

"So you can only feel good about yourself if you lower your expectations?" Clarissa asked.

"It's not necessarily lowering that I should have said, in hindsight," I responded. "It's about setting expectations that are achievable and realistic. At one point, I wanted to be a traveling country-folk-rock singer and guitar player. So I was taken aback when a choir teacher asked me to stop letting noise leave my mouth and just mouth the words so the audience wouldn't be disturbed by my singing during our concert. Pretty soon after that, I figured out that I really couldn't sing and had almost no musical talent. The teacher wasn't being mean. She was right, but I had to evaluate for myself to determine if she was right. I figured out it would be foolish for me to pursue a musical career. So I had to figure out what talents and skills God gave me that I could use and be happy—and that I really had. It took a while to figure it out. Once I figured out what's possible, I set interim goals to see if I was making any progress. A funny thing happened, though. Nothing I dreamed about came true, but I realized after some time that my work still led me to a place where I was content and even sometimes happy."

"So if I'm thinking that the only way I can be useful is to be a Navy Seal like Sarah, what would be an interim goal?" Clarissa questioned. "Like what are you talking about is, I guess, what I'm asking?"

"If you want to be a Navy Seal, it would be really frustrating to have that as your only goal, because you won't be satisfied with yourself unless you've already achieved your goal. But if you're doing well academically, building your fitness, gaining weapons skills, you can have a sense of interim accomplishment," I suggested. "And who knows, maybe you'll change your mind later, but you'll have developed skills that help you do something else."

"I'm not sure I get you. I mean, this just sounds like a bunch of guidance counselor garbage or the type of stuff my dad would say," Clarissa stated.

"Clarissa, I'm impressed with anyone who even considers wanting to be a Navy Seal or any other member of our military," I replied, starting to reach for her hand before thinking better of it.

"So maybe think of it this way. If your ultimate goal is to be a Navy Seal, and a good one, then you have to set goals for yourself. What do you need to do this week, this month, this year? Then celebrate with yourself when you make that happen. And don't take the easy way out of not preparing at all for what you want to achieve, so you risk losing nothing if it doesn't work out. Work at what you want, evaluate yourself fairly on whether you have the skill set to be successful, and then be proud of your effort if you gave it your best. At the end of the day, if you turn out to not have the physical stamina to be a Navy Seal, but you've trained hard to get as close as you possibly can, then you've won simply by proving your ability to work hard."

We'd been talking for a long time at this point. The rain was softening, enough that we could get going again. Clarissa began to stand up.

"Wait," I said. "Read the last couple of sentences, then I'll close this up and we can go."

She pulled the display back up and put her head down to read.

"When I look back now, I'm glad I decided to give life another chance. I've learned that even if you don't always get exactly what you want, something will eventually work out if you make an effort to change," I wrote at the end of that 1986 column. "Even with the efforts I put in to change, life has had plenty of ups and downs. Sometimes it seems like more downs than ups. But at least there are the good times. Maybe that's why (the student's) death bothered me so much. There are no good times in dying."

{ 6 }

Just Shut Up

I GAVE CLARISSA THE LIP CLIP BACK and asked her again if she would record more of her thoughts. She agreed, but this time, only if I gave her my glasses so she could capture herself on video as well. She walked with my glasses pointed toward her, in semi-permanent selfie mode as she roamed out of my earshot.

"So what am I thinking about this? Really, I was thinking you still aren't just letting me think," Clarissa began.

"I got you out of the pouring rain, so all I wanted was a little gratitude and then for you to just shut up and leave me alone. It's not like suddenly I decided I don't want to die. But I don't want an audience. I needed to figure out how and when I could get rid of you so I can stop feeling so worthless, and unwanted and just . . . and just . . . lost. That's what I'm struggling with.

"Then you spout this philosophical bit about maybe Grandpa sent you to see me and fate brought our lives together and golly, isn't the world a wonderful place of magical mystery. I mean, seriously. What a load of crap. At least, that's what I was thinking when you started talking about it. I don't even like the whole idea of fate because if life is all fate, then why bother doing anything. If it's just going to happen, then I'm just a passenger in my own life. Does that make any sense? If life is all determined by fate and my life is miserable, that would mean that God wants me to be miserable. That just doesn't seem right, does it? Would a God who is supposed to be all loving want people to be miserable, or want to pick on me? I kind of liked what you said about having to make choices and that, while bad things have happened to me, it's up to me to decide what to make out of it or how to react. If I don't want Billy and his friends to hurt me, I just have to decide I don't care what they think and it won't hurt as bad. I mean, I don't care, because they're jerks. But I let them bother me anyway, particularly Billy. Maybe if everyone else hated him, I wouldn't care. But what's wrong with me that everyone else likes him and I totally hate him? I don't know. It seems easy to say that you don't care what other people think but I really wish people liked me. I don't want people to make fun of me. I don't want people to pick on me. I want people to like me.

Isn't that normal? I could just say, well that's fate, but I don't believe in fate so it must be that something's wrong with me, right?"

"Your mind has to just be bizarre, Mike. I mean who else would come up with the idea that it's good for trees to be crapped on and that means it's good for people to be shit on. It's like that saying about 'what doesn't kill you makes you stronger,' but what do you do when you're shit on so much that everything stinks and you literally want to kill yourself? You can't get stronger if you're dead, can you? No. I don't know though. Maybe what I'm dealing with is preparing me for something greater and I just can't see it yet. Is that what you're trying to tell me?

"I'm not sure I get what you mean about not living a life of envy. I don't want to be these other people who pick on me all the time. Who would want to be that kind of person who would do that to someone else? I'd hate myself if I acted like that. So, it's not like I want to be some of these other kids. I just want to be happier. I just don't want to hurt anymore. I just want to feel like I matter. I just want someone, anyone, to make me feel like they care without just using me. Is that really too much to ask? Would I feel this bad if I was prettier, or smarter, or funnier or I had a talent that was better than everyone else? Can't I just feel like a real person? Please. That's what I want."

"I have to tell you, Mike, since I'm betting that you're going to listen to this, that when I figured out that you had a Lifelink and geo-mapping applications that would have gotten you out of here without any of my help, I was freakin' furious at first. You lied to me and I'm so sick of people lying to me and telling me they're my friends and then hurting me. Do you know how many boys have just used me? Well, I guess it's not that many, but that's not the point. You didn't need me for anything.

"I was so ready to just get up and walk away and leave you, and then you pull out your old newspaper article. It's convenient that you had that with you. I have to admit, it did convince me that maybe you had been depressed and maybe you did think about killing yourself, but there's no way you were as serious about it as I was. I mean, I have a spear I could've used at the end of my stick and I wouldn't have even considered using it. A bullet is way better. It doesn't hurt as bad or as long and it's more certain to work. So if you were really serious, not just crying out for attention, why use a knife if other stuff isn't gonna hurt as bad?

"What coulda been so bad in your life anyway? I mean look at you. You're old. You're retired a long time. You said you did your dream work for many years. You've got a family and friends. What do I have? I don't have anything. I don't have friends. I don't have a boyfriend. My family doesn't care about me. I don't even like being around me. I mean, I don't want to be alone and you're not alone and I am, so how can you possibly have ever wanted to kill yourself? That doesn't even make sense."

By the time Clarissa handed back the clip and glasses, I was already dealing with the consequences of trying to walk without a good view of where I was going.

Falling Down

EVEN WITH BOTH HIKING STICKS to help me, getting back from Clarissa's rest spot to the main trail was no easy feat, made all the more difficult by my dramatically reduced vision. The rain-soaked ground offered considerably loosened footing, a concept I hadn't even considered when Clarissa suggested the rain was easing enough for us to continue. As tired as I was, I knew she had to be exhausted.

There are few feelings as energy draining as deep depression. In the midst of a depression bout, I remembered that even the simplest of tasks took an enormous amount of concentration and energy to complete. When I compounded depression with weight gain and sleep-deprivation, I felt like I was living life with a giant rubber band around my waist, always holding me back from getting done what otherwise might have been possible.

Clarissa turned to check on me several times as we walked, giving a soft smile or slight wave each time to let me know she hadn't forgotten me as she recorded her thoughts. With the main trail back in sight, she turned just in time to see one of my feet in the air above my head and my hiking poles leaned back at a forty-five-degree angle. My other foot was still in contact with the ground and my back arched as far as it could bend without simply snapping. I tried muscling my way through the fall, lifting one pole out of the ground to move back under me, but it was too late and my muscles had deteriorated from a poor starting point anyway. I was going down.

This wasn't an elegant fall, the type I would occasionally make in my younger years while cross-country skiing, landing in a soft, snow-padded flatland cushion. This was the type of flailing, turning, spindling collapse that made epic failure highlight reels when caught on camera. The twisting face plant into a mud pile, with a follow-up slide down another ten feet of mountainside made it look all the more spectacular, I'm sure. I tried leaping back to my feet to pretend the fall never happened but my body refused to cooperate.

A very soft "Eeeehhhhhhhhhhhhh" was the only sound I recall making.

Clarissa ran toward me, asking if I was okay, but I couldn't get any words out. She began to panic, realizing she left her Lifelink at home and couldn't call anyone for help. At some point before I could get oxygen back to my lungs, she realized that my Lifelink was her best hope for help. She wiped the mud off my finger to get a clean print to open the Lifelink, but couldn't break into the code-protected pocket to get the Lifelink out.

By then, I figured out that I'd had the wind knocked out of me and would likely soon breathe again. Clarissa checked my pulse to be sure I was alive and then yelled for me to follow her finger with my eyes so she could be sure I was conscious. That was easy enough to do, though it had to be quite a sight with my eyes poking through all the mud splattered around my face.

Finally, I mustered enough energy to move my arm and hold up my thumb to let her know I was okay. Moments later, enough oxygen returned that I could breathe audibly. After several minutes of oxygen recharge, I finally spoke. "I'm okay," I said. "Wind knocked out."

Clarissa relaxed.

"Give me your passcode for your pocket. We need to call for help," she said in a tone both urgent and directive.

As she said this, I sat up. I checked my arms. They seemed fine. Wiggled my legs. Felt like I had control. Then I rolled up on my knees, gathering strength to stand back up.

"What are you doing?" she yelled.

"I'm okay," I responded. "If I can get to the trail, I'll be fine the rest of the way down."

"You're as stubborn an old man as my grandpa was," she said. "At least let me help you."

"There you go with the old man bit again," I said. "And here I am falling to show you're right. Frustrating. Just frustrating."

"Sorry, Mike. I didn't mean to call you old again," Clarissa said, before adding with a wry smile: "Even if you kind of are."

She pulled her baseball cap off for a moment to expose an odd assortment of frizzles and kinks, before straightening and re-twisting her hair underneath her cap.

"That's okay. I know I'm getting old. I just don't always want to admit it," I muttered.

It took only a few minutes to walk the rest of the way to the trail with my sight fully restored. Clarissa walked on my downhill side, keeping her hand on my elbow in case I needed additional support.

"Well, that ought to bruise up pretty well," I exclaimed for no particular reason except that I knew it was true.

Clarissa worried whether I could take the rest of the hike down to the end of the trail and out to the main lot. It was still more than an hour away, so I opened the code lock in my backpack, took out my Lifelink device and handed it to Clarissa.

"If I do something stupid from here down, this will open with just my fingerprint. It won't even require proof of life," I said trying to lighten the mood.

"Very funny," Clarissa responded. "Very funny."

For the next ten or fifteen or maybe twenty minutes, we walked fairly quietly. I was concentrating on my footing, trying to make sure I didn't fall again. I was also doing a mental inventory of body parts to be sure everything was working the way it should. I'd pissed myself a little when I fell, but the rain and mud had masked this, saving me from the embarrassment of explaining what happens as body function control deteriorates when we age.

Once I felt comfortable that I was going to be okay, I refocused on what really mattered; making sure Clarissa regained a will to live. I couldn't figure out how to jump back into that conversation at first, so I focused on how I would know that Clarissa was getting better.

"Clarissa," I finally said. "I promised you I wouldn't talk about what happened up here as long as I know you are going to be okay."

"I don't want to talk about it anymore. It's embarrassing," Clarissa responded, so meekly that I had to think for a minute to be sure I heard her right.

"It's not embarrassing," I finally responded while thinking through how to tell her that depression is no more a reason for embarrassment than getting pneumonia. "Embarrassing is falling flat on your stomach and pissing yourself in front of other people, like I just did."

"You pissed yourself?" she asked, smiling and starting to look to see if she could tell before pulling her eyes away as I'm sure the thought of even looking that direction created internal revolt. Instead, she started to laugh. I told her it was okay to laugh, though the soreness in my ribs cut my own laughter short. "It wasn't just my wind that was knocked out on the fall," I added, still chuckling lightly at the ridiculousness of the thought. Clarissa couldn't help but smile a bit more.

"If you want to really laugh, I'll tell you a story about crapping myself in the woods during soccer practice when I was in eighth grade," I told her, "convincing everyone I had fallen in a pile of dog manure by wiping some of it on the outside of my shorts and being driven home with my crap-stained backside sticking out the back of our family's station wagon."

"Oh, that's just gross," she said, mixing laughter and a gag-reflex as she walked.

"You want to hear more embarrassing stories? I have hundreds of them if you want to understand true embarrassment."

"No, no, no. Please stop," she begged. "TMI."

"TMI?"

"Too much information. Seriously, how old are you?" she asked.

"I've heard that before, just not in a while," I responded. "Anyway, back to my question you're working so hard to deflect. How can I know that you're going to be okay? If I don't know this, I think I have to talk to your parents to make sure you get whatever help you need."

Clarissa's light mood quickly darkened again. "My parents don't need to know anything. They'd be embarrassed with me. And angry."

"First, I think they'd be so worried that embarrassment wouldn't even be a consideration. Second, who's going to help you?" I asked.

"I don't know. Who helped you?" she questioned.

I took a few more steps, feeling my age more than ever from the combination of falling and being reminded by Clarissa that I was old.

I thought for several minutes before responding. "In reality, a lot of people made a difference, people I worked with, people who became friends and some of their parents, but I think my biggest breakthrough came during a church youth group retreat."

For the remainder of our hike down, I talked about traveling to a retreat center on Lake Geneva in Wisconsin with a group of high school students, including my nearest brother and sister. I had long since stopped regular church attendance, avoiding discipline at home by saying I was attending services that no one else in the family would be at and providing the same answer to the question my mother asked after every suspected ditching. "What was the sermon about?" Mom would inevitably ask. "Something about needing more money for something," I would always respond, an answer that was most likely at least partially true.

Perhaps knowing I was skipping out regularly and having found a pot stash in the pick holder in my guitar case, my mom insisted that I attend this youth group retreat. I finally gave in, figuring it was a chance to get high in the woods and take a few days off work. I was sure to pack my duffel with enough pot, rolling papers and a lighter to last the long weekend.

"Something funny happened that weekend, though," I told Clarissa. "I found a sense of community, a small group that accepted me, that made me feel I had some worth. I'll never forget the youth group leaders—Deacon Stan and his wife Gay, and Jim and Sharon—for helping me and really everyone else feel a true sense of worth. So, if you're worried about talking to someone who would need to report it to the government health system, are there any priests or whatever religion you are that you can talk to?"

We were nearing the lot where I had parked my rented vehicle. In fact we had it within sight.

"This group you felt accepted you. I thought I had that once," Clarissa offered behind an expression of wistful resignation, gently shaking her head.

"Can you tell me what happened?" I asked.

"I guess, but I'm too tired to talk now," she replied.

"What about tomorrow? I'm calling off my Grand Canyon hike tomorrow on account of bruising and exhaustion. Can we meet somewhere?"

"Well, I don't know. I guess," Clarissa finally relented. "Are you sure you're going to be up to moving tomorrow?"

I gave Clarissa my contact information. She told me hers and I put it into my Lifelink, hoping the information was real. Clarissa rejected my offer to drive her home, saying she had made it up to the trailhead on her own and could get home just fine without any help. I suspected she wanted to be sure I didn't meet anyone I could talk to about her or perhaps was still uncomfortable being confined in a vehicle with a stranger and no Lifelink to communicate out or be traced. Either way, I didn't want to push it too far. Besides, I knew enough about her that I was confident I could track her down if she seemed in danger.

Clarissa promised to message me the next morning to decide where to meet. Most importantly, she gave me the six bullets from the rifle. I could only hope she didn't have any more in a pocket and wouldn't shove the spear into her chest. It's probably just as well she didn't want a ride. It would have been uncomfortable for both of us, particularly for her getting in a car with a stranger.

The trailhead lot was largely empty, just a couple of cars left. Thanks to my slowness, the rain and my fall, we were likely the last people leaving that day.

Normally when I press a hike to nearly sunset, it's because I stopped too often to admire the glistening of a stream, the play of nearby small animals or distant large ones, or the splendor of the entire panorama. After meeting Clarissa, I barely noticed the surrounding environment. I'm sure it was as enthralling as always. Given my concerns for Clarissa, absorbing those views simply no longer mattered.

The vehicles still in the lot had to have brought people camping overnight. If Clarissa lived around

Flagstaff, as she said she did, she could be home in an hour or two moving at a fast pace.

Before getting into my car, I gave Clarissa one last hug.

"Thank you for saving me," I told her.

"Saving you?" she asked with eyebrows raised. "I'm not sure that's exactly what happened."

"I'll explain why it's true when I see you tomorrow," I offered, then slowly and a bit painfully slid down into the seat and headed to a nearby motel. I hoped I had given her enough reason to be curious about why she saved me that she would want to be sure to live until tomorrow.

{ 8 }

Watching the Fall

BEFORE DEPARTING, I ASKED Clarissa to record her thoughts on the last part of our hike and send them to me when she got back home. In part, I wanted to know what she thought but I also wanted to make sure she got home safely. Here's what she eventually sent:

"Oh my God. It was hilarious. I mean, like, hilarious.

"But I felt like a total jerk, because I realized it probably hurt. You didn't just slide down. You went down. Really, it was colossal. Even at my worst . . . you know . . . when my legs felt like detachable stilts, I never fell like that. Sure, I got tripped and pushed and fell plenty of times, but . . . you know . . . nothing as funny as that.

"I guess it would have been funnier if you weren't a nice guy, or so old. If it'd been someone my age, everyone would laugh hysterically, especially the way you spun over and face planted and slid and all that. I guess I just want you to know I'm sorry I laughed.

"I really did start to freak. My mom always says things happen in threes, so after Grandpa and Sarah I'm supposed to be number three to put an end to all this. If you're number three, then I can't do it, or I start another whole group of three.

"Then, after awhile, we started talking about more serious things and how you got help and started to not feel as bad. I guess it's good to know it can get better. I just feel like I've been stuck feeling this bad for so long and it keeps getting worse and I want to know if there really is any hope it will ever get better for me. It's nice to think it doesn't have to stay this way but, really, I guess, it's kinda hard to believe. I don't want to be delusional about being able to be happy and then feeling even worse when it doesn't happen. Aren't I just better off accepting my life is gonna suck, and I just have to deal with it? Well . . . that's not turning out really well, is it?

"Just so you know, I didn't want a ride home because I needed more time to think. We did a lot of talking, probably as much as I've done all year, and I don't really know how I feel about it. Besides, do I really know you? You can't really know someone that fast, and no one I know even knows you exist. If I coulda known for sure you would either take me home or just kill me, maybe, but I didn't want to risk the other options.

"And I need time to think. I mean. That's the main reason," Clarissa said on her recording.

It looked like she had showered and changed before videotaping that message. I hadn't realized she had really long hair, but it was cleaned up and straightened out, falling well below her shoulders. What made me really happy as I played this latest message was that she smiled several times. She probably has no idea how pretty she is when she smiles.

On the walls behind Clarissa I could see a picture frame on the nightstand next to her bed that displayed rotating images. I froze a series of frames and zoomed in to look at the pictures. One image looked like it could have been her grandfather. I copied the picture into my files and started searching for obituaries or news stories about a murdered old man to check the photo against. I needed to figure out how to find her someway other than electronically.

9

Five Things

OTHER THAN GETTING UP TWICE in the middle of the night to piss, I had slept for nearly nine hours when my alarm went off to tell me I had an urgent alert. I unclasped the air-injection mask I wear to help minimize the damage of severe sleep apnea, damage that increased and decreased exponentially when my weight crossed the 190-pound threshold.

I sat up, pulled on overly thick glasses still bent and chipped but at least cleaned from the prior day's fall, grasped the Lifelink to open it with my fingerprint and unfolded the thin, screen-like material to see who was urgently trying to get in touch with me. I assumed, at first, it would be my wife since I fell asleep the night before without calling to let her know I had made it back down. She had sent a message, of course; just hadn't marked it urgent after years of dealing with being on opposite travel schedules.

The urgent message was from Clarissa, a quick video clip of her saying she needed to talk and right away. "I thought I'd feel better today, but I might even feel worse," she told me in her message. Then she proposed a time and place to meet. I quickly messaged her back that I would soon be on my way, then pushed my body to move as fast as it could to not keep her waiting.

Clarissa showed up in a taxi. I didn't know it then but Clarissa had purposely set up our meeting to be far enough away from her home that we wouldn't run into anyone who knew her. Besides, few in Flagstaff regularly visit Walnut Canyon National Monument the way most Americans ignore treasures in their home areas. Clarissa didn't have hiking in mind. I was hoping to take the easy thirty-minute hike around the canyon rim simply to help ease aching muscles.

When Clarissa arrived, she asked me to walk with her to a spot to look at some of the ancient cliff dwellings within view of the park.

We talked, or more clearly, Clarissa talked and I listened. I talked too much the day before. That day, Clarissa was ready to tell me what she felt.

Clarissa was close to her grandfather, perhaps explaining her comfort around someone my age. So that loss was tough enough for Clarissa to absorb.

Making it worse was that the police spread word that he had called the local police a series of racial epithets to justify the force they used in taking him down so aggressively that it ended up killing him. Within weeks of returning to school after that incident, Clarissa had effectively lost the only three friends she thought she had because they all thought her family was full of racists. Her parents were both struggling to keep their jobs among accusations that racism infected her whole family.

Even before these charges, Clarissa had long felt isolated. She'd been six feet tall since she was twelve years old and had been ridiculed mercilessly, so much so that she had withdrawn into a shell. Someone had long ago nicknamed her "rattler" because of her long neck and thin, bony body. She said she had worse nicknames but wouldn't tell me more of them then. As time went on, she was called nearly every nasty snake-related appellation by small groups of kids who clearly took amusement in attacking others.

Clarissa said that for years she had tried to ignore people around her, limiting herself to just three friends she felt comfortable around. Dezbah, Catalina and Angela had been her friends for most of the past three years. They had hung out together, shopped together and talked about boys together. But those three had recently decided to ostracize Clarissa, leaving her feeling completely alone. In the four months since that happened, Clarissa said she probably hadn't said more than a dozen words to any other kids. Her grades suffered even though she tried working as hard as ever. She found it impossible to concentrate and she found herself daydreaming as an escape from what felt like a constant heavy burden of self-hate, embarrassment and anger.

"So let me get this straight," I said to Clarissa after listening to her talk for nearly an hour. "You have, or had, three best friends who all decided to desert you because of something they heard your grandfather said."

"Yeah, pretty much."

"They not only didn't defend you, they piled on to attack you because of rumors they heard about some-one else in your family?" I half-stated, half-asked.

"Yep."

"That doesn't sound like real friends to me. Did you ever try to talk to them about it?" I inquired.

"How can I if they won't talk to me? I was probably already an embarrassment since everyone else always thought I was strange and ugly since I wasn't, you know, doing things other girls were doing. Everyone had always thought that my family was wacko because we went on survival training trips and I kinda like military stuff and shooting and everything," Clarissa opined while staring into the distance.

"Have you talked to your parents about this?"

"They have their own problems. We're already odd in our neighborhood. Most of our neighbors have only lived around us for the past five years or so. Do you think people around us are going to have any sympathy with what they've seen reported about us on One World?" Clarissa asked, shrugging her shoulders in a motion I took as the physical equivalent of saying, "Duh."

One World's social media platform successfully aggregated several competing platforms to create a system that works seamlessly with Lifelink devices, becoming the world's largest interaction forum and the only one able to protect its participants from intrusive government data gathering. I use it because all the people I care about use it.

Clarissa was again dressed in baggy, heavy clothes. The prior day, particularly near the top of Humphreys Peak where temperatures only reached the upper 50s at midday with really strong winds making it feel much colder, her clothing made sense. That morning, with temperatures approaching 80 degrees at much lower elevation, her clothing choices seemed bizarre. Even the desert camouflage colors of the sweatpants and sweatshirt didn't fit with the evergreen forests that surround Flagstaff. She was perspiring even more than I was. I was tempted to ask about her clothing choice but didn't want to make her self-conscious.

"So you feel like an outcast. I get that. I get the sense you're naturally introverted like me to start so making new friends probably doesn't come easily, I'm betting," I suggested. "Let me guess. If you need to talk to someone new, I bet you get nervous and self-conscious, immediately assuming that this person isn't going to like you so it's probably better to not even try. You have to force yourself to initiate a conversation. Some people take this as arrogance."

Clarissa bit her upper lip as she considered her response. I looked down and noticed that she seemed to be pinching her thighs and then her upper arm. She stood up and walked over to the rim. As she did, I worried that she might be trying to hurt herself. I pushed off the back of the bench to walk closer to her so I could react if I saw anything unnerving. But she had gone out of her way to get here.

She wouldn't come here to kill herself in front of me, would she?

Finally turning around, Clarissa had the sullen, pained look that I had seen several times the day before. "Why does everyone hate me?" she asked, speaking in an almost resigned tone. "Why do I have to be so repulsive? Why does God have to hate me so much?"

I look a deep breath. I couldn't help myself starting to tear up at seeing her pain. Admittedly, I'm a crier. My daughter used to love staring at me as I watched life transformation shows when she was young, just to be able to call out the moment I started to cry. But tears at seeing someone who deserves it finally having a moment of true joy were far different from that moment: seeing someone with a real inner beauty in the midst of a painful struggle for self worth.

"Ah, Clarissa," I spurted out after finally gaining control of my emotions. "I can guarantee you that everyone doesn't hate you. I know I don't and at least for the time being I'm still part of everyone. And believe me, you're far from repulsive. And I'm not talking about . . . or just talking about . . . or worrying about physical beauty." I took my time saying that one because I didn't want to suggest she wasn't physically an attractive kid, but I also didn't want to suggest that physical beauty beyond being healthy had to be overly important in the grand scheme of life.

"I can tell from just a few hours of talking to you that you have a real humanity to you, a real way of caring about other people," I added. "That's a gift. That's something special about you. You can't take it for granted."

"How can it be a gift if no one likes me and I feel miserable all the time? It's not like this is new. I've felt like shit for so many years I can hardly keep track. It's just that it keeps getting worse and worse," Clarissa responded, speaking again in a very soft voice that required me to concentrate to hear.

I sighed audibly. "I'm going to guess that part of it is age and hormones and all the emotional torment that accompanies middle school and high school years for so many people," I said. "I'm sure I wasn't fully rational those years. Everyone seems to think of high school as the world you're going to live in. That was my fear anyway. But I found out that in the scheme of life, high school is a short blip that doesn't tell you anything about how good or bad your life will be."

"Well, if everyone deals with emotional torment, why does everyone else seem happy except me?" Clarissa asked.

It's a fair question, I thought while staring at sheer cliffs with evergreens seeming to protrude out of nothing more than rock. I was hoping to find inspiration. Failing to acquire any, I told her what I've learned through the years.

"Look, I'm not an expert in this or anything, but one thing I learned way after high school is that not everyone was as happy as they seemed," I said. "Sure, some people find their comfort zone at an early age and that's great for them. But there's even more who struggle to find their identity in life. At fifteen, I sure didn't have any idea what I would grow up to be, let alone any clue who I was even then. I tried on multiple personalities, sometimes several in the same year— trying to figure out what felt right to me. Every failure, and there were plenty of failures like the time I had the most hideous perm to try looking better, was magnified in my mind. Maybe, most importantly, I learned I had to start liking myself, at least a little bit, to make it easier for others to like me. And I had to learn it was possible to ignore the people who made me feel like I didn't have a place in the world. I came to the conclusion that I had to control how I felt, not give that control to others."

After that we walked around the canyon rim for some time in silence. I didn't know what else to say and it was clear Clarissa was deep in thought. I finally went back to sit on a bench, still feeling the aftereffects of my prior-day fall as Clarissa continued to pace. As she walked, I thought about how I could help her understand that she wasn't alone in feeling the way she did. As an introvert, I had gone through many stretches where I thought no one else could really understand me. That feeling of being alone, that emptiness, was a quick path to despair. What could I do to convince her she wasn't alone?

When she came back to sit, I decided to tell Clarissa a bit more about my background. I would rather have continued to hear about her but she was doing a great job of deflecting my questions and turning them back at me. Besides, I needed to make sure she understood that her pain didn't have to be a lifetime sentence if she was willing to work on it and, hopefully, even get some help.

As I talked about feelings from my youth, I tried to understand them myself. Logically, and certainly in hindsight, those feelings just don't make any sense. Look at all that I would have missed. But during those months, and at times through the years, logic didn't matter.

It took me a long time to understand that depression isn't logical. It doesn't make sense. And you can't just wish it away. Some people have brain chemistry that makes every emotion that much more challenging to manage than for others. For me, getting heavy, out of shape, sleep-deprived and drug- or alcohol-tainted added stress to already terrible feelings of self-doubt and self-hatred.

I can't tell you exactly why I was depressed; it seemed at the time that there were too many reasons to count. I hated being the small kid. For years, some other kids had enjoyed pushing me around, asserting physical dominance as kids and far-too-many abusive adults seem drawn to do to so many people. In retrospect, it was really only a handful of kids who picked on me and not even all that often, but it was enough that I felt safer being alone than being around many other people.

I wasn't comfortable that I had a purpose in life, or could possibly have a happy life. I know my mom really wanted one of her boys to be a priest but I just couldn't imagine that as a life for me. I liked girls even if they didn't have any interest in me the way I wanted them to be interested in me. Sure, some seemed to think I was the little brother friend type at that age. A few were only friendly, it seemed, so I wouldn't hide my answers during tests. Rejection frightened me. Fear of inadequacy manifested itself in so many ways.

As much as one of my favorite memories was of watching Bob Love, Norm Van Lier, Jerry Sloan and the rest of the Chicago Bulls play basketball as a child, a rare family trip to a Chicago Bulls game at the old Chicago Stadium turned out to have a lasting ego-deflating impact. Prior to that game, I thought I was normal. Short and scrawny, sure—and not yet at puberty at the time. But otherwise normal. Then, standing in the open pit urinal at halftime, I noticed the old black guy next to me. He was standing there proudly, not even using his hands to keep from spraying himself. He didn't need to. I mean, my arm was barely that big. I lost all physical confidence that day. I figured every other boy was equipped like him and God had cheated me as punishment for all of my weaknesses and failings. Like Clarissa thought about herself, I decided that God must have hated me to the point he mocked and ridiculed me with what he gave me for a body. It simply wasn't fair. As I was starting to tell Clarissa this, I realized I was repeating a stereotype and an inappropriate topic to discuss with a young girl in any case, but it was true, and enough of it was out of my mouth before I stopped myself that I think she figured out my point anyway.

I decided to quickly change direction.

"How about I tell you about the night I came closest," I said. "Then you can help me figure out why I felt that way. I still don't know that I truly understand that feeling."

"Okay. That's fair," she responded.

"I was in my sophomore year of high school, walking home from work at a deli in the small town where I had lived for three-and-a-half years. I took a knife from the deli with me in my backpack, one of those long thin knifes with a sharp pointy end that could puncture whatever it struck quickly. You read about some of this yesterday, so let me get to the point," I offered.

"I grew a lot after my freshman year, so was almost average sized for my age at that point. I couldn't lay claim to anything exceptional. I wasn't the shortest, or fastest, or most artistic, or smartest or anything. There was nothing interesting about me. I wasn't even the best at being miserable. I wasn't abused at home. I had never starved. I hadn't had to fight through a fatal disease. I was just a blob in the middle, incapable of doing anything that mattered to me or anyone else.

"I think I put up a good pretense most days. I'm not sure most people knew how unhappy I was. I didn't want them to know so I put on a mask. I wasn't often honest with myself and I certainly wasn't honest with people around me, at least when it came to how I felt. My grades started to slip, but even slipping they stayed decent. I could finish all of my homework during classes and still hear enough in the lectures that I never needed to study. I didn't realize how lucky I was that it came so easily. I took it for granted, the way most people who are depressed think everyone else shares all of their best attributes, but no one else has any of our failings. I saw being reasonably smart as a handicap, something other kids ridiculed, rather than appreciating it as a gift," I continued.

"So enough about me. Let me ask you to do something. I want you to write a message and send it to me with five things about yourself that you like. And I'm going to send you a message at the same time with five things I already see in you that are special. Don't send yours though until we're both ready to go."

I started typing almost immediately. I looked up to see Clarissa looking at me, still not having typed anything.

"I can't think of anything," Clarissa finally blurted out.

"I already have more than five, so you have to come up with at least five," I told her, trying to sound encouraging. "Even if it's something as simple as one I might write about myself, like 'my nose hairs trim easily.'"

"That's just gross."

"Yeah, maybe, but it's better than having hard-to-trim nose hairs, isn't it? Seriously, just five things you like about yourself."

It took almost twenty minutes before Clarissa finally was ready to send her list to me. She clicked to send at the same time I did. By then, my list had grown.

I opened up Clarissa's list and read it. "Not a bad shooter, not scared of the outdoors, not mean to everyone, not totally hideous, not totally dumb."

Meanwhile, she read my list: "wants to serve, thinks of others first, deeply introspective, smart, touch of sass, tall, physically fit, engaging smile (when she uses it), enjoys nature, independent, risk-taker, clever."

Both of us bit our lips, though for different reasons.

"Clarissa, you listed all the things you're not. How about putting those descriptions in positive terms, like good shooter, loves outdoors, nice to people, attractive, smart? You can see these in yourself, can't you?" I asked.

Clarissa was still looking down at the ground, sitting on the bench with her elbows on her knees and her hands covering her face. Eventually she nodded while still covering her face with her hands. I took that as a positive sign. Not wanting to push it, I sat patiently, waiting for Clarissa to talk next. It was tough for me to sit there. I still had so much to say.

I looked up at the sky, watching the few clouds overhead move at about my jogging pace. A Cooper's hawk hovered overhead flying in a circular pattern, with other prey-seeking birds within view. A coyote ambled outside the tree line nearby, spotted us and turned back into the woods. I had planned to hike part of the Grand Canyon today, but clearly was fortunate to find a remarkable area to enjoy nature. It was quiet enough I could hear myself breathe.

Finally, Clarissa spoke: "Do you really think these things on your list are true?"

"Of course," I replied. "It didn't take very long for me to see so much good in you, did it? If I knew you better, I bet I could come up with a much longer list."

"I don't know that I think all of these are good things," she continued. "Deeply introspective. Why do you think I'm so miserable? It'd be so much easier if I didn't care about what I did wrong."

"That's reasonable," I responded. "But here's why I think it's a positive. And keep in mind that our greatest strengths are often also our greatest weaknesses. So, someone with confidence—a positive trait—can at times turn overly confident and even arrogant. But I think introspection is a good trait. It means we evaluate ourselves and figure out what we can do better, how we can better behave, what we want to change and improve. This positive becomes a weakness when we let introspection paralyze us, focus us only on what we are unhappy with and lose sight of what makes us valuable to the world."

"What about risk-taker? Why is that a good thing?" she asked, her face again buried in her hands.

"The greatest payoffs in life often come from our greatest risks. Not reckless, thoughtless risks, but risks nonetheless. You took a risk coming here today. You took a risk helping me down the trail yesterday. And I can tell from some of the other things you've told me about your life that you aren't living life in total fear. That's a good thing. But, keep in mind, this strength can turn into a weakness when you're careless," I said.

We sat in silence for a few minutes before I asked Clarissa to record her thoughts again. She wandered off on another trail for a while, taping what's in the next chapter, before returning to sit next to me on the bench. If I had heard her message before the subsequent events happened, I might have better understood what I was about to endure.

10

Breaking Me Down

D WELLINGS CARVED INTO THE CLIFF walls behind Clarissa—one-time family homes that appear to be no more than recesses in massive rock walls from a distance—reminded me that surface perspectives are so frequently misleading in nature. Such is the case with people as well. In hindsight, it would have been good listen to her recording as she was talking, but at least Clarissa chose a visually interesting location as her backdrop.

"Last night," she began, "I guess I was acting too happy because it freaked my dad out and he asked me what was going on. I tried to tell him nothing over and over and over and he wouldn't just leave me alone, so I finally told him I'd met an older man who figured out how to make me feel good for a change. God was that a mistake. He must have cornered me and asked me a hundred questions and he just wouldn't leave me alone.

I just wanted him to leave me alone so I could think. I slammed my door and locked him out and he still sat there bugging me through the door. I don't even know really what I said to finally make him go away.

"I was thinking about you and being on the mountain and how maybe God doesn't hate me as much as I thought, because if he truly hated me, wouldn't he have just let me go ahead and pull the trigger? But then when I woke up, I realized that maybe I had it all wrong and you were wrong. Maybe God hates me so much he doesn't want my suffering to end and so maybe you were sent to make sure I'd be miserable. But then, that doesn't make sense because I actually wasn't miserable at the end yesterday. I mean, I actually laughed, and no one made fun of me and I was in the mountains, so it was a good day until my dad wouldn't leave me alone. Maybe it freaked him out that I was actually happy."

Clarissa paused for a while here, with a soft breeze the only noise captured on the recording for sixty seconds or so. As she looked up toward the sky, I studied the scenery behind Clarissa, noticing that a patch of trees was obscuring another group of cliff dwellings I had initially missed.

"I wonder if he's thinking I might be on drugs because he probably hasn't seen me that way in so long," Clarissa finally continued. "But when I woke up today,

I felt as bad as I did yesterday and that wasn't going to have a good ending if I hadn't met you so I thought maybe I should talk to you again. It all sounds normal when you say it but it's like nothing applies to me.

"I'm not an awful, horrible person so it shouldn't be that hard to feel good, should it? Other people who I think are pretty bad people don't seem to have a problem being happy. I know I make people angry sometimes so I know I'm not perfect. My parents are always furious when I take off and don't tell them but being alone is my only relief. I'd rather go over to hang out with real friends than be alone, right, but there isn't anyone who wants me around anymore. They won't even tell me how I can fix it. They just don't invite me and don't even talk to me or want to even be seen with me and even at school I just feel like I'm trapped on a raft in the middle of a massive cesspool and I can't find the shoreline. I'm just floating in the middle of nowhere and all I want is to be picked up and taken away.

"The thing I keep thinking about is when you said you weren't even the best at being the worst. There's something about that really. You know, when it's so bad you feel miserable but your life isn't so obviously bad that people feel sorry for you. They can't see how bad you feel—or can they see it and just don't care? You don't even get any sympathy for your misery from anyone. I have things other people don't have, some of them good, and people who seem like they have it way worse off appear like they can be happy anyway. I don't get how that happens. If I was beaten or raped or abandoned, I'd be really pissed about it. Maybe I need something truly awful to happen to me to feel better. Maybe if I feel what deep misery is like, life won't seem like it sucks as bad."

Clarissa paused for a long time after that last statement. I could hear her footsteps and see her movement as she paced back onto the trail. Several birds chirped, whistled and warbled in the background. She moved further and further away from the cliff dwellings until I could no longer distinguish them from the rock face.

Minutes seemed to have passed before she finished: "Well, that doesn't make any sense. I mean, who should want to wish to have an awful-er life to feel better? Is that what you're trying to tell me?"

It wasn't too long after Clarissa returned from capturing her thoughts by the cliff that our interaction took a sharp turn.

{ 11 }

Creep Factor

W E WERE FAR FROM DONE talking about Clarissa's strengths when she leaned over and gave me a sweet, gentle hug. As she did, a loud, deep male voice yelled out, "Police, freeze." Three police cars came flying up to the edge of the Rim Trail. A helicopter flew overhead with a sharpshooter latched onto its edge aiming a weapon toward us or, more accurately, toward me.

I tried lifting my hands in the air but my left arm went numb. I was hoping it was my pinched nerve acting up. It didn't feel the same.

I hunched over the bench, not sure what I was feeling but certain it wasn't good when I heard her voice next.

"Daaaddd!" Clarissa yelled in an intensity and harsh voice I hadn't yet heard while waving aggressively to try to get the police to back off. "What the fuck?"

Clarissa's father was running our direction. Police surrounded me, yelling at me to get my hands in the air. I tried as best I could to raise both hands but apparently wasn't quick enough. I was thrown the rest of the way to the ground with my face pushed down.

"Who is this pervert?" John Coleman yelled at Clarissa.

"What are you talking about?" she screamed back in an even louder voice than I thought she could muster.

"This is the man?" John yelled quizzically as I turned my head to look at him.

About then, the police rolled me over with my hands cuffed behind my back. I was too stunned to say anything or to even move.

"Stop it. Stop it. Stop it!" Clarissa kept yelling. "What is going on?"

One of the officers looked at John Coleman.

"Is this the man sleeping with your daughter?"

Clarissa unleashed at least a half dozen strong rights and lefts into her father's gut before the police could grab her and restrain her.

"This is the 'older man' you came here to meet and the man you spent all day yesterday with?" John asked Clarissa.

"What has he done to you? Did he rape you?" one of the officers asked Clarissa.

"Oh, gross," she replied to the officer before turning to look at me. "He's like my grandpa's age."

"So why'd you tell me you were meeting an older man who told you he could help make you happy? You told me it's the first time you'd been touched that it didn't hurt," John asked his daughter. "And I found these in your room," he added, holding up a set of condoms.

Clarissa put her head down to her knees, with her hands behind her head. "I hate you, Dad. I hate you. I hate you. I hate you!" she yelled, both fists moving up and down to accentuate each use of hate. "Those condoms get taped to my locker every day with nasty notes. Did you even bother to read the hate notes in the box under them?"

"Well, what are you doing with him?" John asked.

"You don't want to know," Clarissa replied, still screaming loudly and sternly.

"Yes, I do want to know. I'm panicked about you. I don't have any idea what's happening with you. I feel like I've lost my little girl," John said in only slightly lower-volume voice. "What's he doing to you?"

One of the officers took Clarissa's Lifelink and started to scroll through her messages. He opened the last message, the one I sent her that listed her positive attributes. After reading it, he began to grill me.

"Why would you send a fifteen-year-old girl a message that talked about her sass and her smile? I think I know what that's code for. And you talk about her serving you and being physically fit. Clearly, there's something physical going on here and you're not leaving here until you admit it," the officer barked.

I just shook my head, still trying to figure out what was happening and too startled to speak.

"Did you know she's fifteen years old?" he asked.

"Yes, I believe I know how old she is," I responded, slowly and quietly. "But there's no law against talking to a teenager in Arizona, is there?"

"This is all the evidence we need with the visual confirmation of physical contact between the two of you to make an arrest," the officer said. "The officer who has been watching you today reported that you were starting to engage in sexual activity with the girl."

"You're all disgusting. He was not," Clarissa yelled. "I hugged him. What is wrong with you people?"

"Put her in a car and tell her to shut up," one of the officers yelled, after which Clarissa was grabbed and pulled over to the back seat of a car by one of the officers. John Coleman started to follow before turning back toward me: "If I find out you did anything to my daughter, I'll take care of you myself."

Gathering every ounce of energy I could, I spurted out: "You might want to worry a little more about helping your daughter."

"What's that mean?" John asked.

"I think it's better if Clarissa tells you," I said before the pain from being thrown onto my sore ribs became too much and I passed out.

When I regained consciousness, I was in a local hospital, with an IV feed in my arm, a heart monitor beeping next to me and oxygen tubes attached to my nose. It took a bit for me to get my bearings and realize where I was. I checked and realized that I didn't have any handcuffs or other restraints on me. I found the control to the bed, using it to lift my upper body so I could look around at my surroundings. I could see to the doorway. No sign of a police officer outside the door. Maybe they've figured it out by now. Maybe Clarissa told them.

After a while I rang for a nurse to get me some water. Instead a police officer entered. "The parents have decided to not pursue any charges against you," the officer told me, "and I need you to sign this release acknowledging that you agree." I was still a bit dazed and my glasses even more chipped than they had been the day before, but I read through the release and figured out pretty quickly that I was really agreeing to not sue local police for false arrest and the injuries I suffered at their hands. I signed anyway. Life was too short to pursue a court case.

John Coleman came in next with a quick apology.

"I'm so sorry for what we did," John told me after he re-introduced himself. "You have to understand that Clarissa just has been in such a deep funk and then she comes home acting even more strange and almost happy. Now that I understand, I'm so grateful that you are taking time for her, for Clarissa."

"She's really a remarkable young lady," I told him. "You should be proud of her, and you should let her know that you're proud of her."

"I wish I was always proud of her but sometimes she just scares the hell out of me," John replied. "She hasn't listened to a damn thing I've said lately."

"But, even then, you always love her and care for her?" I asked.

"Of course."

"So make sure she knows."

"She knows," John claimed.

"Don't be so sure," I suggested.

Not long after John walked out, Clarissa came in, tensed up from what appeared a mix of anger and sadness.

"I can't believe they did this to you . . . that the police did this to you . . . that my dad did this to you," Clarissa said, her cheeks quivering as she spoke.

"Don't be mad at your dad or the police," I replied. "He might have overreacted, but that's what parents do sometimes. I can't say I would have done anything differently if I only knew what he probably knew, so I'm not upset with your dad at all."

"But they hurt you."

"Just physically," I said. "More importantly, how are you? I take it you told your parents how we met."

"Mostly."

"What does mostly mean?"

"It means I told them I was really bummed out and I started talking to you, and you are helping me be less bummed out."

"So . . . the rifle?"

"I'm not going to tell them that," she replied. "They would stick me in a mental hospital or something. But I explained your message and everything so everyone realizes that arresting you was just stupid."

"So your parents don't really know how bad things are for you?" I asked.

"Well, I didn't think so, but I guess they've been really worried. I just kept shutting them down whenever they tried to talk to me. I didn't think they could understand, or would even care," Clarissa responded.

As she talked, I noticed that Clarissa looked different. She was still wearing baggy pants, but she had on a long-sleeve concert T-shirt for some band that performs in a way that I refuse to acknowledge as music. At least the baggy sweats weren't an everyday uniform. Her reddish brown hair wasn't rolled up inside a baseball hat, though the high ponytail she wore still kept her lengthy, slightly frizzled hair away from her face. She smiled just a bit more as we spoke, though was clearly upset at how I had been treated and constantly asked me if I was okay. I'd been able to get a sense that she felt better about herself, certainly better than when I first encountered her. We'd made some progress with Clarissa.

It was only a matter of hours before they would let me out so I thanked Clarissa for visiting and told her I would let her know when I was mobile again.

An hour later, Clarissa's father was back at the entrance to my hospital room.

"Do you mind if I come in?" he called out from the hallway.

"Of course not."

"I wanted to tell you again how badly I feel about having misjudged what was going on," John said. "And I'll understand if you're too angry to be willing but I really need your help."

"Help?" I asked. "What can I do?"

I pointed to the chair next to the bed to suggest that John sit down. He ambled his hulking frame, pulled out a handkerchief to wipe sweat from his forehead and took a seat.

"I'm really scared for Clarissa," John said. "She's my baby girl and now I'm not going to be able to sleep without having nightmares of waking to find her hanging or OD'd in her bedroom. I've tried to talk to her about her mood before but she doesn't want to talk and the harder I push, the more she pulls away. She's just been so unhappy and, these last few months, she's just isolated herself more and more."

Several of my medical tubes had recently been removed so I sat up on the bed to look at John, pulling the blanket over my lap.

"Clarissa tells me she told you what we've been talking about," I said.

"Yeah. I'm not surprised at how she feels," John replied. "But I'm more panicked than ever."

"I see that, and I have to say, you're right to be worried from what I've seen."

"Yeah."

"So tell me. What's changed about Clarissa that has you worried the most? Who is she when she's happy?" I asked.

"Oh my God," John said, his face lighting up. Even his disheveled eyebrows seemed to straighten as he talked about Clarissa. "She's my little girl, my buddy. Our two older girls are more girlie-girls. Clarissa always did things with me. She was the first to want in on anything we could do together—hiking, fishing, shooting, fixing things up, even yard work. And she's so good at it. She's just a natural. Wherever I went since she was little, I could always count on having Clarissa by my side to help."

"And you've lost that connection?"

"Yeah, especially since my dad's death. She's just almost empty these last few months and I feel like she's hiding from me and her grades are falling apart. And Cara, my wife Cara, isn't having any better luck. Clarissa just disappears for hours and hours and sometimes even whole days. And she's getting better at keeping us from tracking her."

"John, I'm going to do my best to help you. It's pretty clear to me that Clarissa's got a great heart, a real concern for other people, but just can't seem to recognize everything, or maybe even anything, that's good about her," I said. "And I get the sense that she's taking an extraordinary amount of abuse at school from some of the kids there. Has she ever talked to you about that?"

"I've tried to ask her but she just won't tell me. Like I won't understand," John responded.

"I wonder if she's just worried that acknowledging feelings is a sign of weakness. Was she always the tough kid?"

"Yeah, I guess. She always was driven to just plow through whatever obstacle was in her way. She'd get cut and not even stop until someone else noticed her bleeding," John said. "But I don't think of her really as tough because she was always so gentle with anything helpless. She just worried about everyone else first and never worried about herself or her own safety for that matter."

"What do you mean, her own safety?" I asked.

"That girl, Clarissa, has scared the bejeezus out of me from the first day she could crawl. She thinks she's invincible sometimes."

"She's done the same to me already and I've only known her a couple of days," I noted.

"What do you mean?"

"You know, I'm afraid that she's just not afraid. That's probably as much as I can say without breaking her confidence. You know enough to know that she needs help, right?" I asked.

"Yeah. I can see that now."

"Before I forget, Clarissa mentioned something about notes where you found those condoms," I noted.

John's face turned red, likely from the embarrassment of having misinterpreted what those condoms signaled.

"Yeah."

"Did you read those notes?"

"No, I don't want to invade her privacy and make things worse between us," John stated.

"I think we're past the point where privacy issues should be your primary concern, don't you?" I asked.

He looked at me for several seconds before nodding his head up and down. "I guess so."

"So why don't you go home, tell Clarissa you want to read the notes she mentioned or just find a way to get them, so you can learn a bit more about what she's dealing with? Maybe that will help," I suggested.

"But, if I do that, she might not ever trust me again."

"Remember, she's the one who told you about them. Don't read them to punish her. Read them to help her. You need to be in crisis mode now, don't you think?"

"Yeah, I'm with you on that," John responded.

"So go home and spend some time with her. Don't ask her. Tell her you need her to help you. She seems to respond to people who need her help," I said.

"Yeah, I guess she's always been that way. Always wanting to help other people," John replied. "That might be a good idea. I'll think of something."

At this point, John stood up and came over to shake my hand. John didn't seem like the type who was used to asking for help so I was sure that coming there hadn't been easy for him. But the fact that he cared enough to talk gave me hope.

"One last thought, John," I said as he neared the hallway. "The worse she seems to be getting, the more time you need to spend with her and the more you need to involve her in your life. Don't be so afraid of saying the wrong thing and setting her off that you stop trying."

Grand Addictions

MY FAMILY TRIED TO CONVINCE ME to just come home. I had at least three offers to pay the rebooking fee to move my departure up early but I planned this trip to last four more days and I wanted to stick it out. I convinced everyone at home to calm down; I was fine and would be home soon enough anyway.

After being finally released, I took a taxi to my motel. It's the kind of place a cheapskate like me stays in when traveling on my own, though I've stayed in places where I wore socks into the shower and slept fully clothed to minimize contact with anything in the room. This motel was better than that but you could still tell that whoever cleans these rooms didn't do so with a great deal of pride.

Regardless, when I finally made it back to my room, I wasn't worried about any of this. Physically, I was more beaten than I had been in a decade. Even the walks to the taxi at the hospital and from the taxi to my room had been tough. I'd been prescribed medical marijuana for the pain, a prescription I'd filled before giving it much thought. The other options were all opiates—more addictive drugs than pot—so I opted for the marijuana.

As I sat in the motel room, I debated whether I really needed it. I had quit cold turkey before my sixteenth birthday, a vow to myself I had broken only twice in college. People tell me marijuana isn't addictive and that may be true for some people. But what was addictive to me was how good—or, at the time, how much less bad—it felt to be high. The problem with pot for me was not that it generally sucked to use it. The problem was that it generally sucked to stop, but getting high killed my initiative and drive to work for anything lasting more than a few minutes or hours. It was a cheap short-term physical crutch that only masked my ongoing internal pain.

I was fortunate to avoid the deadly long-term consequences that follow on a path to addiction for many. It took a while for me to figure it out but lasting personal satisfaction takes a long time to build and seems to only come with real sacrifice for the vast majority of us. It's hard work and many days come and go without the payoff for staying on a narrow path.

Suicide Escape

I don't have a particular problem with medical marijuana for other people who truly need it, though not for the people who say they need it because they get bummed out when they run out of weed. But, for me, I knew I couldn't start down that path again.

Anyway, I got back to the room and decided to try getting by on aspirin. Fortunately, I was exhausted enough to fall asleep fairly quickly. By the time I awoke, a dozen messages awaited, all with the purpose of checking on me. Four were from my wife, two from Clarissa and one from John Coleman, who apologized again for what happened.

Rather than respond directly, I updated my One World status so anyone trying to contact me would know that I planned to be up and moving the next day.

That was the plan anyway but when the next day came, I was still too sore to move. After that initial nap, I hadn't slept well, tossing and turning as one sharp twinge after another shot into me whenever I tried to move. I stared over at the package of joints and fought my desire to use them. The temptation was gnawing at me; practically begging me to light up. What more did I think I was going to accomplish in my life, I asked myself, that I couldn't just give in to easing my pain? But I knew if I started, I wouldn't be able to stop.

Put a one-pound bag of chocolate-covered almonds in front of me when I'm hungry and watch to see if I can eat just one. Unless I'm completely full, the odds are against the bag's contents lasting long. When I try even this simple exercise in self-control, my hand will stuff candy in my mouth as if responding to magnetic attraction. Soon enough, the bag is empty.

I did get in touch with a few people on One World. Even short discussions were tiring so I pulled on my apnea mask and slept as much through the day and night as possible.

Waking the following day, I felt better. Not fully functional, mind you. But better.

It was time to head to the Grand Canyon. I sent a message that I was up and good for the day and heading out for a hike. I invited John and Clarissa to join me if they were interested.

John responded quickly that he would like to go with me but needed to be at work. He added that he would wake Clarissa to see if she wanted to come.

I'd returned from the next-door convenience store with my yogurt and coffee for breakfast and waters, nuts and dried fruit for the hike when Clarissa responded that she'd be happy to go with, even sending me her home address to pick her up on the way. I was sure she agreed out of guilt for my arrest but was happy she agreed nonetheless.

As we headed to the first overlook in the Grand Canyon, Clarissa and I had the chance to talk some more. She fidgeted around; checking every pocket, cup holder and seam in the car. I hadn't contemplated this possibility in advance, so was caught unprepared when she pulled out the medical marijuana package as I took a final drink of coffee.

"Well I guess the arrest wasn't all bad. Looks like you got some free weed out of it," she said as she opened the package and started counting how many joints were inside. She looked back at the carton label. "You didn't smoke any yet?" she half stated, half asked.

"No and I'm trying not to smoke them. It's not for me," I replied.

"Then, can I have them?" she asked.

"I don't think that's a good idea," I responded. "Do you get high? Do you take other drugs?"

"Not really drugs, but since you have some and you're not going to use it, what harm is there? I mean, it's government approved weed so it's got to be safe."

"Safe is a relative term, Clarissa," I said, thinking I was going to have to make the transition from friend to disciplinary adult if she didn't back away.

"Still, other kids are always talking about how fun it is to get high," Clarissa said as she pleaded for me to let her take them. "It might be something I can start doing with people . . . you know . . . friends."

I breathed heavily as I tried to think of what to say next. To say I felt in an awkward place is a bit of an understatement. "Imagine me making this call to your father . . ." I started to say.

"You can't call my dad on this," she responded in a tone that made clear her righteous indignation.

"I didn't say I was going to. I was saying imagine if I had to make the following call to your dad: 'Uhhh, John, this is Mike. I've got bad news. It turns out that it was a mistake to let Clarissa get high before we set off hiking trails along the cliff faces around the Grand Canyon. Turns out that when you lose a little control out here, it can have deadly consequences,'" I told her.

"Oh, that's ridiculous. I'm not saying that I need to get totally high. I'm just saying that I want to try a little. And you have a bunch that you're not using," Clarissa pleaded.

"Look, there are some things in life that are better to not try, because they have consequences that aren't worth the risk. You might be one of the people who can smoke the occasional joint and not let it affect your life. But you might also be one of those people who aren't physically or mentally predisposed to handle it. What do you do then?" I asked. "I told you about how drugs and alcohol contributed to my failures and my depression. Why would you want to add that risk for yourself, especially now?"

"Oh, you're so starting to sound like a parent."

"Besides, Clarissa, can you imagine what the police in Flagstaff would do to me if they find out this old man is passing out joints to fifteen-year-old girls? That arrest might not go quite as well for me," I commented in trying to ease the tension.

"Yeah, I guess that might not look so good for you, when everybody's already a little suspicious of you anyway," Clarissa said.

"Suspicious of me?"

"Well, I mean, because of the other day," she noted.

As we entered the park, we pulled over to the side so we could watch elk nibbling at the grasses surrounding an evergreen forest plateau. As we did, several cow elk took turns searching the surroundings, making sure no one approached their calves too closely. At times, the elk would lift their heads up to yank off leaves on some of the deciduous trees mixed in amidst the evergreens.

From there, we continued to the first overlook. The canyon walls were infused with rich ambers, rusts and tans in alternating stripes. Trees shot out of small inlets sometimes hundreds of feet removed from the next nearest signs of life with trunks that start out perpendicular to the cliffs and curve to end up parallel at the top. Some canyon areas were dotted with green vegetation, while others were barren except for the millennia-old tapered cliffs.

A few of these stops later, we were parked within range of the path I wanted to take down to the Colorado River. Clarissa didn't mind that hiking down halfway was as much as I thought I could handle; not that the hike down would be so rough, but that getting back to the top could be a struggle and I didn't want to be too far removed from help if I needed it.

During certain parts of the hike down the canyon walls, you forget all about the surrounding beauty, focusing on making sure your feet are on firm ground before taking the next step. The path narrows at various points, twisting, bumping and turning around the canyon walls. Every once in a while, someone gets moving too quickly, thinking they can stop their feet from moving forward just because they want to stop before realizing that gravity has a stronger hold on their body than they might desire.

It was while walking these paths that Clarissa became a more complete picture for me. I wish I could recall all of what she said in vivid detail but the reality is I was distracted watching my steps.

When we finally made it to a ridge overlook about halfway down the trail, we sat for a while to talk, hydrate and eat.

"It's great that you had a chance to connect with someone as heroic as Sarah," I said after I caught my breath, drank several large gulps of water and opened a bag of mixed dried fruit and nuts for us to share. "Most people go through life without meeting anyone who we all think of as a hero. So what did you take from meeting her? From what I've read, she was a pretty remarkable woman."

"What you've read is probably true. I guess what I was amazed by is that she took time to search for someone like me when I was lost and even took time to come out to my watch spot and talk to me. She didn't have to do that," Clarissa responded.

"So, if I'm hearing you right, you're telling me she really cared about other people and was a risk taker, clearly. And she had to be physically fit," I stated.

"Oh, yeah, definitely."

"And she had to be independent, in the sense that she pulled off a remarkable feat on her own."

"Yep, that's her."

"Would you say she was smart or clever?"

"Both."

"Hmmmm. I'm trying to think of someone else I know who I've used those words to describe. Oh, let me check my messages," I said as I opened my Lifelink to display and turned a message toward Clarissa. "There it is. The message that nearly got me in boiling water with the local police."

"Yeah. I know you say that but I haven't done anything close to as cool as what Sarah did. I don't know that I could even do it and I don't want to be a failure by not being able to be as good as Sarah."

"Whether you can be 'as good' as Sarah isn't relevant," I replied. "What matters is whether you are as good as Clarissa. There are all types of heroic people and heroic actions. Do you think parents who sacrifice for their families aren't heroic? How about people who go to jobs they don't like to create a better life for people around them? Is a singer not a success if he doesn't become a superstar or an engineer not a success if she doesn't invent great products, even though they made the world a better place through their work, their volunteering, their friendship and everything else they contribute to the world?"

"Yeah, yeah, yeah, I've heard that type of stuff from you already. That's your thing about trees mattering even if animals are crapping on them. I don't want to be shit on my whole life. I want to be someone people admire and respect. If I'm going to live, it has to be for something more than this lousy life."

"Clarissa," I responded. "Everybody gets crapped on. It's as inevitable to life as animals pissing at tree trunks or birds crapping on trees. It's what we do about it that matters. We can either let it bother us, get annoyed and dispirited and angry, or shake it off, let the crap and piss fall to the ground, and use it as fertilizer to grow and become the best person possible."

Clarissa looked at me a bit stunned for a few minutes: "That's the first time I've ever had someone tell me I should be happy that people are shitting on me."

"That's not exactly what I meant," I replied. "All I'm saying is that you can use whatever you have to endure to strengthen yourself instead of giving in to it. I'm not excusing abusive people or inviting painful experiences. I'm just saying that bad things happen to everybody. Even people you think have a perfect life have tough things happen to them. The people who succeed over a long life take those difficulties and use them as motivation or lessons or whatever to help grow. I think it's important to think about every failure or pain and figure out if there was a purpose to it; something I can better handle or do to help others because of what I learned."

We sat quietly side-by-side for a while, neither of us looking at the other. I wanted to give her time to think. But I realized that I hadn't really been complete in what I had said so I interrupted the quiet. "Clarissa, it's great to want something more. I encourage you to be the best person you possibly can be, to work hard, to realize you'll fail sometimes and get back up and keep working at it," I said. "But at the end of the day, you have to define success for yourself. You have to figure out how you can live a life that makes you happy while respecting the rights of others to live lives that make them happy."

I'm not sure Clarissa was really listening to me as I said this. So much of this is true but it sounds trite and contrived and preachy and wholly lacking in promising Clarissa that she can just decide what she wants to achieve and it will happen. "I know I'm boring you so can I tell one of the strange points in my life when I realized I had achieved one of my life's dreams without even knowing it?" I asked.

"Sure. Why not?" Clarissa relented.

"When I was a little boy, I told you my family used to go camping at this place out in a rural part of Illinois. My parents had bought a small plot of land there and we'd go out on weekends in our tents and pop-up camper and just run around in the woods for hours and hours. Sometimes, I would lie down on one of trees that fell over a creek or sit by the shore of a nearby lake and just dream of the day I would grow up and be rich and have a massive backyard with woods and lakes and hiking trails, chasing squirrels and seeing deer running and riding bikes on roads and trails. I figured I needed fifty or one hundred acres of land to have the backyard I wanted."

"I'm not sure where this is going but it would be cool to have a lot of land to myself," Clarissa offered.

I nodded agreement and continued. "When I first got out of college and started earning enough that food money didn't run out a day or two before the next paycheck, I looked at what it cost to own that much land in the Washington, D.C., area I lived in at the time. There was no way I could ever earn that much, so I put that dream aside. But I hiked in the mountains and ran and biked in local forests most nice weekends and found my connection with nature."

As I was talking, we both sat near the cliff's edge, looking down at the Colorado River. I was clearly more afraid of heights than Clarissa, whose knees were bent with her feet hanging over the rock edge. The breeze blew our hair back away from our faces. Actually, the breeze blew Clarissa's hair back away from her face. Even combed fully forward, my hair barely reached the top of my forehead. I stopped talking for a minute, leaning forward to make sure Clarissa could hear me and was still listening.

"So that's your achievement?" she asked in clear sardonic tone.

"No. Not quite anyway. Then we had kids and, after awhile, we were so busy that I stopped taking the kids on Sunday morning hikes in the woods. I lost my connection with nature and part of me felt empty. When my kids stopped playing traveling sports and at least a portion of my weekends became my own again, I found an arboretum just a few miles away from my home. Suddenly, I had the backyard I always dreamed of— seventeen hundred acres of woods and lakes and trails, and, even more, friendly people to talk to on occasion. I realized after going there for more than a year that I had managed to achieve one of my childhood dreams. I didn't achieve it the way I thought I would achieve it but my dream had been fulfilled. That's what life is like. You struggle and push and go off path. You get frustrated and angry at times and then, one day, you see someone or accomplish something where you just go, 'Oh, that's what all of this led me to.' If you get too dead-set on a single outcome, you might not even see that the good you end up with was worth the struggle."

"So you had a good life. Good for you. But how do I know my life will be worth it to me?" Clarissa asked.

"There's no guarantee," I acknowledged. "That's for sure. Except that I can guarantee that when you give up, when you stop trying, when you let addictions control you, the outcome won't be what you want."

We'd rested enough at that point and it was time to start heading back up. The early afternoon sun was beating down hard. I'd missed a few spots on the back of my neck with sunscreen and I could feel them burning. Even with sunscreen coated on now, I had another pain to distract me from still sore bruised ribs.

When our hiking took us around a canyon wall where we lost exposure to the wind, the heat quickly became unbearable. I sweated almost as fast as I could consume water. Clarissa was absolutely soaked, having hiked wearing thick, loose sweat clothes. Just before we sat down to rest, she had pulled off her sweatshirt to reveal another dark, long-sleeved T-shirt with symbols on it I couldn't decipher. She stuffed her sweatshirt in her backpack.

We stopped for another quick rest in a shaded spot, giving me time to drink more of my third liter of water for the day and to share more of the fruit and nuts. When I stood up to start moving again, Clarissa looked at me, clearly wanting to say something to me, but unable to force the words out of her mouth.

I looked at her for a second or two before realizing she was frozen. "Just spit it out," I said. "Whatever it is, it can't be that bad."

Finally, she relented. "I'm boiling hot so you're going to see this when I take my sweats off so I'm just going to show you," Clarissa said using the meeker voice that stole her vocal cords during her moments of deep discomfort.

Standing in front of me, she began to pull down her sweatpants. I turned my head sharply to avoid looking and heard multiple bones crack in my neck.

"I have shorts on," she assured me. "That's not what you're going to notice."

"Okay," I said as I turned back to look at her. As I spotted what she knew I would see, I put my fist over my mouth, clamping my lips tightly between my thumb and index finger. I tried to contain my reaction but moisture soon cluttered my vision. I swallowed a bit of my own vomit so Clarissa wouldn't see the full level of my disgust. After a minute or two, I pulled off my glasses and wiped away tears with the inside of my sleeves, then clasped my hands in front of me and bowed my head into them.

The inside and outside of Clarissa's thighs were thoroughly bruised, likely from the pinching I had noticed days earlier. Even worse, she had razor slash marks all over the inside of her thighs at various points of healing, several of which seemed to be fresh wounds.

"And you may as well see this too," she told me, turning to face away from me and pulling up the back of her shirt to reveal more cuts and bruising around the sides of her bone-protruding ribs.

I could hardly stand to see this any more.

"There's more," she said, "on my arms, where no one can see under my sleeves."

"Did someone else do this to you?" I asked, knowing that no response could be satisfactory. Part of me hoped that abuse could explain the marks and her depression, if we could get her out of the abusive environment.

"No," Clarissa admitted or at least stated. "I do this to myself when I need a relief from hurting."

"So you hurt yourself to reduce how much you are in pain," I said, not quite knowing what to make of this since I was never a big fan of pain.

"I guess so," she replied.

I knew for certain then Clarissa needed more help than I could provide and I wasn't going to be around much longer in any case.

"Do you know why you do it?" I asked as we continued our hike upward. We had covered a few S curves upward before she responded.

"It makes me feel better, at least for awhile," she finally admitted, before accelerating to get well ahead of me. When hikers approached coming down, Clarissa would take off her backpack and hold it in front of her thighs until the hikers passed. That told me she wasn't hurting herself to draw attention she clearly needed. Finally, I caught up with her and asked her what she meant about this making her feel better. "You know, it tells me that I'm at least alive, I guess, and maybe I kind of feel like I deserve to be in pain," she said. "Did you ever do anything like this?" she asked.

"No, I don't think so. But you have to remember that depression hits people differently. Those of us who face it all respond in different ways. I buried mine inside and then climbed out the basement window after everyone was asleep and walked the streets for hours, often getting high, but sometimes just thinking and trying to get the world to make sense to me."

"Did you ever get it to make sense?" Clarissa asked.

"That's a really good question," I responded, trying to buy time to think. "Not really. I guess what I finally concluded is that it didn't make sense, that life isn't fair but that it wasn't good for me to compete to see if I could absorb more misery than anyone else. But hey, to your hurting yourself question, I can only recall one stretch where I did it regularly, though it wasn't out of depression."

"Well that's odd."

"Well, I'm certainly not normal the way people think of normal, so I'm okay with being odd," I said, hoping I could lighten the mood enough to make Clarissa feel okay with sharing how she had hurt herself.

"So what was it?" she asked.

"In grad school, I had a cost accounting class. None of it made any sense to me. I used to study in our dining room. Sometimes, in the middle of studying, I would stand up, turn around and just start banging my head into the wall—over and over and over."

"Why would you do that?" she asked.

"I was hoping that maybe my brain was just out of place and if I banged it hard enough, it would eventually make sense," I said, looking down to watch my feet as the path narrowed. I walked directly behind Clarissa to avoid being too close to the edge.

"Did it work?"

"Actually, what happened is I finally figured out that debits and credits worked almost the opposite of what logically made sense. Once I realized that the language was purposely constructed to not make sense to normal people, I could understand how it worked," I replied. I knew my story had nothing to do with Clarissa's cutting and pinching, but I was trying to make her feel comfortable discussing her behavior.

"So it made sense because you figured out it didn't make sense?" Clarissa asked.

"That's the best way to describe it," I acknowledged.

"That makes no sense."

"Of course not," I agreed as I turned to get in front of Clarissa and look at her. "But back to you, Clarissa, if we can figure out someone you can talk to who can help you feel okay without hurting yourself, would you be willing to talk to them?"

"Yeah I guess," she replied in the soft, withdrawn voice she used when it was clear she was uncertain about herself. "I guess as long as it doesn't have to be reported."

It was a good time for a break so we took out our Lifelinks and searched the area for counselors, mental health professionals, clergy and others who might specialize in teen depression. Our search was made more difficult by needing to keep Clarissa's case from being reported, but we ended up with several options.

Not wanting to wait, we made an appointment for Clarissa to see a counselor the following week. Clarissa agreed to tell her parents she was going to see someone for help.

The hike up took almost twice as long. I needed to stop regularly on the way up and I could tell Clarissa was getting frustrated with my slow pace. I offered to let her just go ahead and wait at the top but she always stayed within eyesight of me. We didn't talk much the rest of the hike up. I tried to convince her to take the lip clip microphone and try explaining to me why she hurt herself but she said she was too ashamed to talk about it and couldn't entirely figure out why she did it anyway.

"Doesn't it hurt?" I asked her as we approached the top.

"Of course it hurts, and it's so stupid," Clarissa said. "But I just can't help myself. It's like I lose control of my hands and I'm cutting or pinching before I know I'm even doing it."

"Do you think you can stop?" I asked, holding the lip clip toward her in one more attempt to convince her to tape herself.

"Don't you think I would have stopped by now if I knew how to get myself to stop?" Clarissa asked. "I feel like an alien in my own body sometimes." I gave up trying to pull anything more from her. I don't know much about this behavior or what causes it. So I focused on finishing the hike and heading back to Flagstaff.

I got out of the car briefly when we reached the Coleman home to talk to John and meet Clarissa's mother Cara. They seemed like good people who cared about their three daughters and their community. John, clearly the talker in that relationship, told me that the only good fortune of my arrest at Walnut Canyon was that he had been able to talk to the local police captain about rumors spread by his officers about racism inside the Coleman home. He wasn't wholly satisfied with the response but at least they had made progress toward resolving their lingering dispute.

I'd said goodbye to Clarissa quickly that day. I know she had to have regretted her decision to spend a whole day with me. But I was grateful she went.

Getting back into the car, I felt another painful twinge. I decided I couldn't put it off any longer and set my destination for the hospital. Then it was my turn to deal with an issue I'd purposely ignored the last three weeks. I knew that I wouldn't be able to ignore it any longer when a doctor came into my room accompanied by an official government health representative.

Both introduced themselves to me. Before they could tell me what they came to tell me, I started with my questions.

"What stage is it?" I asked.

"You knew?" the doctor responded.

"I noticed it a few weeks ago," I told them. "I came out here for a week of hiking to try to decide what to do about it. Even if treatable, I wasn't sure I wanted to bother. But now, I think I have to at least try."

Non-Hodgkins lymphoma runs in the family. Over the years, it has killed my dad and numerous other relatives. Strangely, even in-laws have been killed by the same disease so when I felt a cherry-sized lump under my armpit, I had a good idea of what I faced. Treatment has improved substantially from what some of them endured, but I knew it would be a long time before I ever hiked the outdoors again and I might not ever have the strength again.

After putting myself officially on the waiting list to begin treatment, I messaged Clarissa to let her know I was heading home to get treatment for a lump I had discovered.

"What does that mean?" Clarissa messaged back.

"Well, when I told you that you saved me, Clarissa, this is what I was talking about. Meeting you convinced me I needed to put aside how depressed and angry I was at the thought of having to face this cancer and so I'm going to fight it. I'd been thinking about just letting it go. After all, I've already lived a lot longer than I expected or really even had a right to live."

"You have cancer?" she asked in a message.

"So it seems," I replied.

It might not have been the right decision to tell Clarissa through a message, but I knew I wouldn't have the heart to tell her otherwise. With as much loss as she's endured in recent months, dealing with another potential loss had to be a rough burden to carry.

After thinking about how poorly I'd handled this, I sent another message: "Clarissa, I know this is tough on you and I won't blame you if you don't want to talk anymore. You've lost so many people in your life lately and I know that getting to know a stranger who might not live long is very uncomfortable. And if you can't handle talking to me, either messaging or video call or whatever, just know that I'll be thinking about you and appreciate what you did for me and praying for the best for you."

A message from Clarissa popped up on my Lifelink that she wanted a video chat.

"You're not a stranger to me," she told me when we finally connected. "You know how to reach me and I know how to reach you."

She looked back to see a big smile on my face.

"Besides, I have two things of yours that I need to return," Clarissa said, with a clear look of guilt on her face as she held up two joints she must have taken. "Should I put them in the mail?"

"I'll just drop by and get them from you on my way to the airport tomorrow," I replied. "Then I can say 'see you later' in person."

{ 13 }

Crapped On Again

"**I** WAS FURIOUS AT YOU AT FIRST for reacting like you did when I showed you my cuts and bruises," Clarissa said in another recording. "The last thing I need is someone else thinking I'm a disgusting pig. Then I realized you weren't upset because of how I looked but because I keep hurting myself. And I guess it really does look gross when I actually look at the scars and cuts in the mirror. It's getting harder and harder to hide it especially now that it's so hot out. I realized I'm pinching all the time, almost an instinctive reaction. The cutting bit is more recent. I still need to be alone to do it because I watch the blood drip for a while too.

"At first, it bothered me how much you talk when we're hiking but I'm kind of getting used to it. You seem to want to hear what I think and it's nice to know someone wants to listen to me. I guess you would be really lonely out there without me, hiking for so many hours without talking to anybody or anything. So it's good to keep you company and to have someone who has the time to talk to me."

Clarissa was sitting far enough back from the camera that I could see her fists wedged against her inner thighs. She was pinching herself again and probably didn't even know it. When she soon moved her arms up to cross in front of her, it was clear how much her unconscious mind controlled her motion.

"I'm kinda mad about how you told me you had cancer. I guess you might be number three after all. Makes me feel awesome really. People meet me. They make me happy. They die. That's my superpower. I kill people. How do I use that to make a better life? So I was in a real deep funk last night.

"Then I realized I think I have you figured out. When you see me feeling bad for something that sucks in my life, you tell me a story about something that sucks in your life or something stupid that makes me think about something else. I wonder if you really even have cancer or you're just telling me that so you can say your life sucks worse than mine and make me feel better. Except that I don't feel better. I feel worse. You seem like a good person and you get cancer but Billy Kunzler can fall drunk off the bleachers and not get a scratch and no one even figures out he's drunk. God I hate him. I know. I know. I have to forget about him, not give him any power over me. Ignore him. Live my life. I hear you. It's just hard to actually do.

"Maybe that's what you mean about life isn't fair and I just have to get over it. But I want life to be fair. Why shouldn't it be fair? But it's not fair. So how do you make it fair? I guess maybe it can't always be fair so, I mean, maybe you're trying to get me to think about what I have that's good more than what I have that's bad or don't have at all. Is that it?

"Anyway, I guess even with the bad news afterward, I'm still glad I went hiking with you. So I was thinking about this and I started to feel guilty about taking your joints. I figured you were going to be really pissed and I'm not sure I should have told you because you might never have known. I still don't get why you are so adamant that you don't want me to start, but I felt terrible anyway. It's got to be better than downing a pint of vodka or whatever else I can find a lot of nights just so I can go to sleep, don't you think? I guess that's one of the things I haven't told you yet. My grandpa had a lot of liquor stashed away and I've been going through it at night sometimes. I know I shouldn't but I'm just doing it to help me sleep.

"Well, anyway, I guess I'll see you soon so I'll tell you in person too but thank you for listening to me and not thinking I'm worthless."

{ 14 }

Departing

SAYING GOODBYE TO CLARISSA was difficult. I didn't know if I would ever see her again and suspected that I might not. But I believed we were both better off for the time we had together.

At first, I exchanged regular messages and calls with Clarissa in the days after I returned home. I spent a lot of time in those first few calls trying to convince her to not drink as a crutch and trying to get her to understand that if she couldn't control her drinking on her own, she would have to stop entirely or have her life ruined.

I was surprised Clarissa hadn't mentioned her drinking earlier given how brave she had been in sharing her feelings but I guess even the most open of us hide aspects of our lives we find embarrassing. She hadn't contemplated the toll drinking was taking on her body and mind—sapping her real sleep, her energy and her health.

To Clarissa, alcohol had just been a coping mechanism, a "friend" to help comfort her. But it became clear her drinking was out of control to the point that this "friend" was beating her upside the head and speed-bagging her gut many mornings.

I guess it's true that it's impossible to really know someone completely. All I could do with Clarissa was try to pull off the disguises to help her figure out what she wanted and, more importantly, what she was capable of doing.

Our video chats helped lift my spirits in the initial months waiting for my tumor- and node-removal surgery. Eventually, I made it to the top of the list. During bed-ridden days in that span, my wife sometimes took my Lifelink mid-discussion and continued conversations with Clarissa outside of my reach, knowing I couldn't detach from the convoluted system of wires and tubes hooked up to and around my body. Clarissa really started to enjoy talking to my wife and soon enough was messaging directly with her as well. All good, I thought. If everything doesn't work out for me, at least Clarissa can stay in touch with her.

As tough as some of those days and nights were enduring treatment, losing what was left of my hair, feeling my muscles shrivel and my bones ache, I felt

Clarissa had been another angel sent to help me find the will to keep fighting. Finding that will wasn't just about Clarissa. It was also about my family and friends, the moments I would miss and the people I would never meet if I didn't fight through it. As I wrote long ago, there are no good times in dying.

My contacts with Clarissa became more irregular as the summer neared end. Once a full load at school added to her aggressive fitness regimen, our contacts became a sporadic response to a status update change or quick message. During these communication lulls, Clarissa's parents were nice enough to keep us in the loop on her progress. I even started talking semi-regularly with Mrs. Coleman, Cara, whom it turns out had been dealing with her own serious depression issues for some time.

Cara was excited to see Clarissa talking about her future. Clarissa had taken a job tied into the survival camp where her friend Sarah had worked. Taking that new role gave Clarissa the chance to earn a substantial income to help pay for college but required her to improve her fitness and her grades. Becoming the youngest member of a team that included ex-military people made the new job appealing and gave Clarissa a source of pride she had been lacking.

With an improved sense of confidence, Clarissa reconciled with some of her old friends. She didn't have as much time to spend with them anymore, but talking through what had angered them gave Clarissa the chance to establish a comfortable peace. It seemed that Clarissa was moving the right direction.

At least for now, I've lost the stamina to go hiking and, I have to admit, losing the independence to pursue one of my favorite activities is a difficult adjustment. But adjust I must. I have no right to feel anything but fortunate for what I have left and for the life I've already lived.

When the weather is nice, I still sit by a lake at the arboretum, looking up at the evergreens towering above the hill on the other side of the lake. My legs can't take me up the hills but I still think of those hikes with Clarissa whenever I sit there and stare at those trees.

Recently, I sat thinking about Clarissa, looking at a picture John sent to me of her at the finishing line in a Halloween obstacle course contest. She wasn't hiding her face. I didn't spot any bruising or cut marks and she was even wearing shorts. She had added what appeared to be a fair amount of toned muscle to her frame and her face wasn't nearly as skeletal as I had recalled. Her nose doesn't even look at all out of place when her face isn't so shrunken.

But what I noticed more than anything was Clarissa's smile. In the moment she crossed that finish line, with arms raised over her head, she radiated a true happiness and pride I had only hoped to see during my days hiking with Clarissa.

It's moments like that, few and far between though they may be at times, that make the struggles of daily life worth enduring. While I was looking at the picture and thinking about Clarissa, an alert came that I had a message from her.

"I just want you to know that I'll never forget what you did for me."

I closed the message and couldn't help myself. I put my head down under my hands, only gathering myself after a kind stranger came to ask me if I was okay.

"Yes, miss," I told the stranger after gathering my breath. "Tears of joy. Tears of joy."

I'm glad I took that hike up to Humphreys Peak.

It's funny. When I left for Arizona, I thought traveling there and hiking up Humphreys trail was my idea.

Now, looking back at all that has occurred, I know better.

Better yet, now I know Clarissa.

{ 15 }

One Day At A Time

WHEN I FINISHED WRITING about our journey together, I asked Clarissa to record one last message describing how she was feeling. I'm so happy she told me it was okay to go ahead and share what she was thinking throughout our journey together, in addition to sending one last message for me to use. Here's what she sent:

"I'd like to tell you that I don't sometimes still hurt. There are days that just suck and I feel like if I could just disappear, I would. But there are more and more days that don't suck and some of the days are even okay, some of them even good. I have a couple of new friends at the fitness center. I don't worry so much about people at school because people who just know me without other people telling them not to like me seem to think I'm okay. It's kind of like a fresh start for new people to get to know who I am, and not who I was or who other people thought I was.

"I realize that not everyone is gonna like me but the most important thing is I'm not disgusted with myself anymore. Some days, I even feel decent about who I am and maybe more important about who I can be when I leave high school. I have a new purpose to my life and can see now that I have a reason to exist that I couldn't see at all when we met.

"It's funny how a few kind words, even from someone who was a stranger at the time, can matter and really make a difference. It did to me.

"I've been thinking about our hikes a lot. I just can't explain it. I mean. I don't know why we met. But nothing that's been good the last few months would have ever happened if we didn't meet. I mean . . . I have a chance to make the world a better place and feel good about myself doing it. That never would have happened if I had . . . if I had . . . if I had pulled the trigger.

"I gotta go. I'm going on a hike back up to Humphreys Peak. This time, though, I know I'm coming back."

Acknowledgments

After writing a story that shares so much personal experience, it's difficult to know where to start in expressing my appreciation. I'll start at the beginning. I would not be the person I've become without my parents. Even amidst the worst of my depression, I never doubted they loved me and wanted me to succeed and be happy. I simply didn't see a path forward. Bernard John Bushman left the world far too soon, yet his lessons remain ingrained nearly two decades after his passing. Lois Mary Bushman improved many lives as a mother and as a pastoral associate at St. Peter's Church in Geneva, Illinois. It's a treat to see her living her life with renewed joy as Mrs. Spognardi.

At various stages of my life, many others have helped me find my worth. Deacon Stan and Gay Szara, along with Jim and Sharon Elgar, led a church youth group I participated in at parental insistence. A retreat weekend they led was a critical turning point in my life. Ken and Betty Collins, along with others, provided adult guidance through times when I needed to hear right and wrong from someone other than my parents.

Mike Bushman

It wasn't until I finished writing this story that I realized that my friends Mike Collins and Dave Steel became part of my life at about the time I began seeing a path toward a future. We've been friends now for thirty-five years and I value that friendship in a way that I find difficult to express even to them.

I also need to particularly thank Carly Jacobson, an amazing friend who shared her personal story in the foreword to this book. My wife and I are fortunate to have worked with Carly and been part of her life. I look forward to working with Carly on her burgeoning C.A.R.L. Project to facilitate the types of discussions on mental health that were so important in Carly's recovery as well as my own.

Of course, I also have to thank everyone who helped make this story better. Over the past year, I've received thoughtful guidance, edits and support from Dick and Shirley Riederer, Bryn Collman Henning, Bill and Cathleen Bushman, Christine Hudzik, Dave and Jennifer Steel, Carly Jacobson and Candice Gardner, Cynthia Kadela, Jennifer Marsh Ginder and many others.

Special thanks also to Tim Benson at timbenson-photography.zenfolio.com for allowing me use of his work on the next page.

I can't do my work without friends and family and am eternally grateful to all.

ABOUT THE AUTHOR

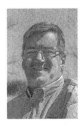

Armed with a BS in journalism from the University of Illinois and an MBA, with honors, from the University of Chicago, Mike Bushman spent twenty-five years working in the interwoven worlds of national and global government, business and the media. Mike's first two novels, *Melting Point 2040* and *Secession 2041*, tell action-suspense stories of a future America segregating toward division. He is currently writing a third novel in that series describing a pathway toward reuniting the nation around a common but politically neglected moral principle.

While set in the same time span as the trilogy and incorporating the character Clarissa Coleman first introduced in *Secession 2041*, *Suicide Escape* is intended to be able to be read and understood independently of those novels. The story focuses on what is, unfortunately, a timeless challenge.

Contact Mike at:

www.mbushman.com

www.facebook.com/AuthorMikeBushman

mike@mbushman.com

Twitter: @m_bushman

Fifty percent of author profits from *Suicide Escape* are being donated to mental health organizations.

Made in the USA
Monee, IL
03 October 2021